Exotic Tails

A Veterinarian's Journey

S T E V E N   B.   M E T Z , D.V.M.

Exotic Tails

A Veterinarian's Journey

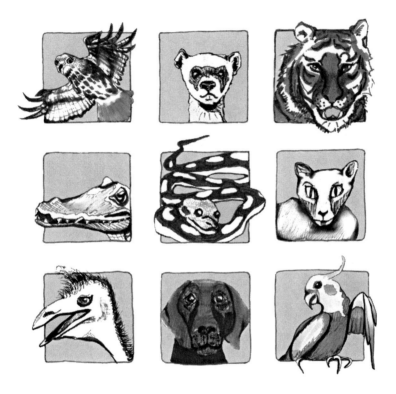

STEVEN B. METZ, D.V.M.

Published by Wind Ridge Publishing, Inc.
Shelburne, Vermont 05482

Exotic Tails
A Veterinarian's Journey

Copyright 2012 by Steven B. Metz, DVM

Cover art by Iona Woolmington

Published by Wind Ridge Publishing, Inc.
P.O. Box 752
Shelburne, Vermont 05482

ISBN: 978-1-935922-13-1
Library of Congress Control Number: 2012941674

This book is dedicated, with respect and love, to my brother,
Dr. Lawrence Metz, who was responsible for my admission
to the Ontario Veterinary College, and thus for my subsequent career.
Because he took my repeated application rejections upon his own shoulders,
he never stopped working on my behalf until my dream was realized.

Contents

Foreword

In August 1985, our family completed the trek from Washington, DC to our new home in Shelburne, Vermont. The station wagon was overloaded with our family of four, assorted bikes, luggage and boxes, and two "inherited" cats that had been abandoned in our old neighborhood in Washington.

One of these two cats was just odd: oddly shaped, oddly colored, and oddly named—Brownie Fox. We knew that as he grew older he had gotten progressively slower afoot, meandering dangerously across busy streets, plodding down sidewalks, and bumping his way through DC's grass alleys; one neighbor had sardonically nicknamed him "Swifty." Brownie Fox had a difficult and anxious trip north in our car, unable to carry out his bodily functions and appearing to be in real discomfort. So when we learned that one of our new neighbors on our road in Shelburne was a small animal veterinarian, we counted our blessings and made a quick appointment to see him at his nearby hospital.

It took Steve Metz about ten seconds to render a stunning verdict: "You realize, of course, that this cat is blind." Despite the abundance of clues, none of us in the old neighborhood—nor, I would add, the local veterinarian—had ever guessed that Brownie Fox was progressively losing his vision. Perhaps he had eaten the wrong meal or experienced another kind of harmful exposure, Steve suggested, and he sent us off with some medication to ease Brownie Fox's understandable distress.

Those words served as our introduction to Steve, who, along with his entire family, has been an important and valued friend to us over these past twenty-seven years—once we eased past the concern that he might view his new neighbors as essentially unobservant dummies.

Over the years, Steve has continued in his professional role as perceptive and trusted veterinarian for our family's pets, including a wide range of assorted felines and a much-beloved Labrador retriever. He would keep us abreast of current cases, and occasionally I would accompany him over the weekend to his hospital to provide a minor assist or simply to observe. Additionally—

and this is described in the book—Steve provided crucial external leadership during my years as chancellor of the Vermont State Colleges, reforming and rebuilding a key college academic program.

We quickly came to appreciate Steve as an extraordinarily knowledgeable and dedicated veterinarian, and also to value his broader understanding of and interest in virtually all dimensions of the natural world. We also have learned from, and been entertained by, his apparently endless supply of fascinating stories about the animals he has tended and the characters he has dealt with—both patients and their owners—as well as about his early dreams and subsequent adventures on the road to becoming a veterinarian.

I was therefore delighted when Steve told us of his plans to write this book, looking forward with eager anticipation to his retelling of many stories I faintly recalled. Upon reading the drafts, however, I realized how much more I was learning than I had previously known about his life, his work, and his insights into the worlds of both domestic and wild animals and their intersections with human society. I also learned that indeed there were plenty of additional stories to enjoy.

Further, speaking as an educator, I realized that this book holds important lessons about learning as a lifelong process and about personal growth—about holding onto cherished dreams and finding creative ways to achieve them despite formidable obstacles, that formal education and training are merely a prelude to a richer education and understanding that can come through experience, and that curiosity and the eagerness to continue to learn will make all the difference over a career and throughout a life.

This is a wonderful, entertaining, and educating book for us all.

—*Charles I. Bunting, former Chancellor, Vermont State Colleges*

Steven B. Metz, d.v.m.

Introduction

It is 2:30 a.m. on a Monday night as I watch a beloved three-and-a-half year old domestic longhaired cat, Buka, lie in an oxygen cage struggling for every breath. His half-hysterical owners are watching both Buka and me, looking for some sign that the medications I have administered are helping, or that some additional action will bring about a reversal of Buka's agony.

The setting is a modern, well-equipped companion animal veterinary hospital in Shelburne, Vermont, in July 2002. I have been a veterinary practitioner for thirty-two years, and although I have not had specialized training in emergency medicine or cardiology, the x-ray films of Buka's chest clearly show the problem. His heart is enlarged and his lungs are full of fluid. He almost certainly has the condition known as dilated cardiomyopathy, and his heart muscle is failing to maintain adequate circulation.

I have given all the indicated medications and put Buka in an oxygen-enriched atmosphere. Nevertheless, as the minutes pass, he continues to gasp for air and his tongue is tinged with bluish-purple color that indicates his bloodstream is not receiving the necessary oxygen. Periodically, he changes his position or his posture in the oxygen cage in an attempt to get more air into his fluid-filled lungs.

"Isn't there anything more you can do?" It is the owners' repeated question, and it is my question too; indeed, that question is the foundation upon which I have built of all of my professional life. I hope the true stories in *Exotic Tails* demonstrate the value of persistence. It has served me well in my journey to become a veterinarian and now, moreover, I hope that persistence has served our faithful animal companions as well.

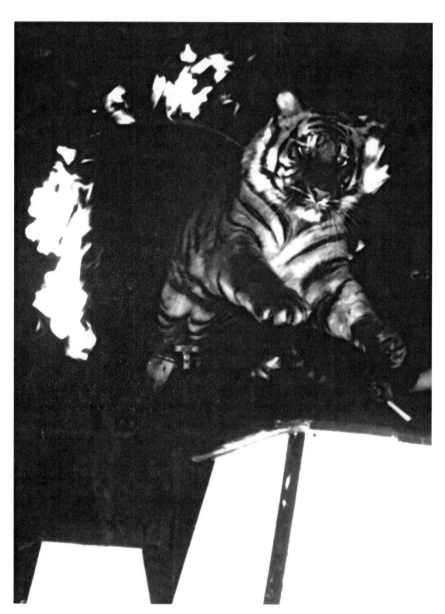

Princess was a Bengal tiger with the Shriners' circus.

chapter one

From Phobia to Pursuit

My road to veterinary medicine was far from conventional: I read every horse and dog story in our local library, but was terrified by close encounters with even the smallest of pets. How, then, did a seven-year-old boy grow to overcome an almost phobic fear of animals? How did he later become a veterinarian that could walk into a zoo enclosure with an unsedated male leopard, or crawl into a circus wagon with a seriously ill Bengal tiger? How did he learn to work with aggressive dogs and swearing cats, or handle coiled boa constrictors sleeping in guitars? The answer lies in a revered grandfather, desperate parents, a wise junior high school science teacher, and a circus clown with a toothache.

My Russian grandfather, Morris Katzman, was a cattle dealer from the "old country." He purchased dairy cattle that were past their prime as milk producers and resold them at a local livestock auction, hoping to make a profit. Western Massachusetts, even in the late 1940s and '50s, was not exactly a thriving agricultural area; however, a surprising number of dairy farms were still operating, and my grandfather seemed to be on a first-name basis with every farm owner. His days consisted of traveling from farm to farm, exchanging banter with the farmers—each telling the other how tough times were and how difficult it was to make a living. The visit culminated with the query, "Well, what have you got to sell me today?" Ninety percent of the time, the answer was a shake of the head—nothing. But on a rare occasion, the farmer wished to sell a cow, and then the fun began. The bargaining, the haggling, the sad stories—each man trying his best to outdo the other. Often my grandfather would break off the discussion and leave the farm, shaking his head and muttering to himself (for all ears to hear) about how unreasonable the farmer was acting. When this happened I was sure that the two parties would never be on speaking terms again. But an hour or two later, or perhaps the next day, back to that farm my grandfather would go to resume the haggling and the storytelling, the whole performance masterfully performed by each party.

As an eight-year-old city boy spending the day with my grandfather, the whole experience was magical. We would pack lunches, get into the salmon-colored 1941 Dodge (that my grandfather insisted "ran like a top"), and take off for the country of western Massachusetts. My grandfather would choose an area and visit several farms on each trip. As he was driving, he would tell stories about each farm or farmer, commenting on the herds, farming methods and abilities, his or her personal character traits, and fascinating information about the animals and the farms.

At lunchtime, my grandfather always managed to find a cool, shady spot to pull off the road. We would stop, have our lunch, and then it was a short nap for my grandfather while I read a book or walked to the edge of the pasture where we were parked. I watched the grazing cows, observed their behavior—their placid cud-chewing and interactions with each other. I would usually pick out a favorite cow, although my criteria were quite inexplicable. Throughout the day I bombarded my grandfather with questions: "What breed of cow was that red and white spotted kind?" "Which breed of dairy cow is the best?" "Why do some cows have no horns?" "What's growing in that field?" "What do cows eat in winter?" What a learning experience for a city boy who otherwise had little to no contact with animals or agriculture! Everything about those days appealed to me—the atmosphere of farmhouses and barns, being outdoors with animals, and learning about a totally foreign lifestyle and culture. Why, I even found the odor of cow manure attractive. Thanks to my grandfather, when my first-year veterinary school professors initially labeled me a "city boy," I surprised them with my knowledge of farms, farm animals, and farming methods.

All this time—and from as early as I can remember—I was absolutely terrified of dogs. Of course, this was well before leash laws were even a dream, and I knew where every dog in the neighborhood lived. My home was only two blocks from my elementary school, but I would not walk to school alone for fear of meeting a dog on the street. There were no school buses at this time, either. To say that my fear was inconvenient for my parents is a gross understatement. To begin with, they could not understand it. I had had no unpleasant encounters, nor were my parents or my older brother afraid of animals. In fact, my father could go up to the crankiest, most unfriendly dog and have the dog kissing him moments later.

So what were my parents to make of the fact that their frightened son constantly pestered them for a family dog? Even when they saw me sit on the floor stroking and talking to the neighbor's gentle old English setter, they could not imagine bringing into our home the very creature of which I was so terrified under most circumstances. My father was a busy dentist with a demanding practice, and my mother had absolutely no background with animals of any kind. My brother was my only ally; we used to spend hours poring over dog books and magazines discussing the merits of various breeds. I wore out our local librarians with requests for all their books on dogs and horses, often reading several per week.

My parents withstood the pressure for a few years, but saw I was not outgrowing my fear. It was seriously affecting my ability to interact with my classmates outside of school. A counselor advised them to get a family dog; therefore, in desperation and with great misgivings they yielded when I was about twelve years old. After much discussion, we decided upon a boxer, due in no small part to an almost weekly encounter with an exceptionally gentle and beautiful dark brindle male, Von by name, who lived not far from our neighborhood.

My mother, in particular, had serious misgivings about our choice, because she thought the breed looked vicious due to the black muzzles and undershot lower jaw. Nonetheless, we began to shop for a puppy, and one holiday weekend in New Britain, Connecticut we found ourselves looking at a pen full of beautiful young boxer puppies. As my mother approached, one of the puppies came over, stood on his hind legs and licked my mother's hand. Bear in mind that my mother was the least enthusiastic about the whole idea. Moreover, she was a fastidious housekeeper. To our surprise, she declared, "This is the one!" The puppy was not a dark brindle like Von, but rather a golden brindle, but we were all so relieved at this first sign of acceptance by my mother that within a few hours we were driving home with this puppy in my lap. He was given the highly imaginative name "Duke."

Duke's arrival caused a total family revolution. All sorts of adjustments needed to be made, mostly by my parents, upon whom the brunt of the serious care fell. At the end of that first long weekend, my father went off to work and my brother and I went to school, leaving my mother to cope with and exercise our young, un-housetrained, energetic puppy. As we got the story from our neighbor and family friend, she spotted my mother walking young Duke up the street with tears streaming down her face. The neighbor called in alarm, "Charlotte, what's the matter? Is someone in the family sick?" My mother cried, "Look what's happened to me. They've all gone and left me with...." The neighbor got my mother calmed down with such remarks as, "Look how handsome he is," and "He really seems to have taken to you!" And the latter observation certainly proved true. Duke became devoted to my mother, to the point where he was her constant companion both in the house and when she went shopping. Years later, when my mother went through a period of major depression, Duke never left her side, sleeping beside her bed and sitting beside her when she ate breakfast. He was a powerful force in her recovery.

As for the twelve-year-old boy too frightened of dogs to walk the two blocks between home and school, I was so eager to come home and be with my dog that I fairly flew home, not noticing any other dogs, but anticipating the greeting I would get as I walked through the door. Regularly, I would be knocked down by the muscular young boxer, rolled over several times, and administered a thorough face washing, football tackling, arm pulling, and other roughhouse tactics. I steadily lost my fear of dogs. After all, went my reasoning, what more could any dog do to me than what I endured at the jaws and paws of my beloved Duke.

Never was fear replaced more surely by understanding than it was in my case. Now I knew what made dogs act and react the way they did: why they jumped and barked, what got them upset, how they responded to different situations. Slowly my confidence grew as I developed a feel for canine behavior that has served me well throughout my career.

My brother and I went to dog shows with Duke; I met and handled hundreds of other dogs, which further grew my confidence and understanding of the dog world. I had actual contact with a veterinarian for the first time when Duke needed vaccinations and other care. Neither Dr. Snow nor his home office was fancy, but I was fascinated with the most minute details of canine health care and easily impressed.

I cannot leave the subject of the entrance of Duke into our family, however, without relating his effect upon my grandfather. In the old country, dogs were workers. In my grandfather's experience, dogs drove the cattle to market. They ate whatever scraps were available and slept in the barn or with the cattle on the road. The idea that dogs were even allowed inside the house, let alone assigned a favorite armchair (Duke appropriated it for his own gradually, and eventually, we all just gave in) was beyond Gramp's understanding. "A dog is a dog!" he would roar in apparent disgust when Duke came over to be patted. Gramp would brush off his trousers and settle back in his chair. Being in his late 70s or early 80s, my grandfather would soon fall asleep and start to snore. Duke would cock his head at the sound, and suddenly sound a loud sharp bark. The rest of

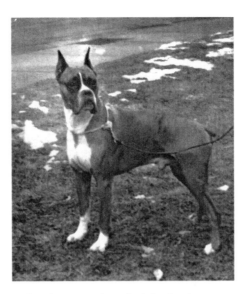

Duke, a boxer, was the author's first family pet.

the family, who observed this drama reenacted several times a week, convulsed with laughter. My grandfather awakened—sometimes it took more than one bark—noticed us all giggling, and sternly commanded Duke to "keep still." It wasn't long, however, before some of us caught Gramp surreptitiously slipping Duke a few pats and ear scratches when he thought nobody was looking. Still, we were constantly reminded, "A dog is a dog."

We didn't hear much about a dog being just a dog, though, when Duke came back from one of his rare stays at a boarding kennel and was in a very thin condition. Homesick, he had refused to eat well and had lost considerable weight. When my grandfather saw our skinny dog, he was enraged with the kennel. Forgotten was the scrap diet his dogs were fed in the old country. The kennel owner was a thief and a murderer! It was more of a task calming Gramp down than putting weight back on Duke.

Lest this turn into a dog story, I will relate one final comment about this canine that exercised such profound influence over my life: My parents kept a picture of Duke in their bedroom after his death and said good night to him every night. In fact, when I began this writing my mother was approaching her ninety-fourth year and still said, "Good night, Duke."

About cats and the many other creatures I would later be called upon to handle, examine, and treat, I remained ignorant until much later in my education. Next I was to acquire a fascination that first became a hobby and later, my professional life.

In September of 1951, I began attending a new school—Forest Park Junior High School. It covered grades seven through nine. My homeroom and science teacher was Miss Claudia Schmidt. When my friends (none of whom, of course, had any firsthand knowledge) heard about this teacher assignment, they groaned with sympathy and predicted a completely miserable year with lots of detention—staying after school to clap erasers and wash blackboards for various crimes and misdemeanors committed throughout the day. However, being fairly stubborn, I decided to determine this myself. It was many months, though, before I began to appreciate, admire, and later revere Miss Claudia Schmidt.

Everyone has a favorite (or villainous) teacher story from his or her school days. Mine involves Miss Claudia Schmidt. She was a spinster in her late 50s or early 60s when I came to know her. She was a type of schoolteacher whom I suspect one doesn't encounter in our schools very often these days. She was quiet, polite to her students, and never raised her voice or lost her dignity, even in the face of extreme provocation which, alas, occurred all too frequently with our age group. She also had an absolutely iron will. If Miss Schmidt said something, we could count on that pronouncement coming to pass.

The subject she taught was Science (with a capital "S"), not physical science, chemical science, nor natural science, but Science. For most of us, as seventh graders, it was our first formal exposure to science and the scientific method. Miss Schmidt taught us to observe and to reason, not merely to learn facts. I can still remember the experiment demonstrating the expansion of metal in response to heat—a simple but dramatic demonstration. She picked two of the most obstreperous students to assist, one to hold a large brass ring with tongs. The second student was to pass a cold brass ball attached to a holding rod through this ring, and then heat the brass ball over a Bunsen burner flame and immediately try again to pass the ball through the ring. Of course, after being heated, the ball had expanded so it would not pass through. The ball was cooled in ice water, which made a very satisfactory sizzling sound, and could then be passed through the ring again.

Miss Schmidt gave each of us a notebook and proceeded to dictate the scientific method of recording our observations. To this day, almost sixty years later, I can remember the exact words upon which she insisted as accurate scientific observation, not supposition or conjecture. This distinction, by the way,

S t e v e n   B .   M e t z ,   D . V . M .

is a key principle in the education of anyone working in the sciences to this day.

In our classroom was an aquarium containing some tadpoles. We were to observe and record weekly in our notebooks the physical changes as the tadpoles matured, thus introducing us to the concept of metamorphosis. Because I had taken up the hobby of keeping tropical fish at home, I volunteered to feed and clean this aquarium, thereby earning the title of "teacher's pet"—a serious charge in those days. To counteract this label, and with the prompting of some of my friends and classmates, I agreed to play an April Fool's joke on Miss Schmidt. I agreed to report the fictitious death of these tadpoles to Miss Schmidt during our first period of the day, thus bringing to an end (at least briefly) the tedious weekly notebook entries.

This undertaking may not seem terribly significant to an adult, but no student of Forest Park Junior High School had ever dared play any type of joke on Miss Claudia Schmidt. It was unthinkable! The only levity in the classroom occurred at Christmas, when Miss Schmidt told us about hearing a "rustling noise" in her chimney only to discover a package of calendars, which she distributed to us as her Christmas present. She told this story with such total solemnity that not a giggle was to be heard in the room (a major exercise in control for seventh grade boys and girls). Now I proposed to announce publicly that her cherished experiment was a failure.

On the morning of April first, I arrived in the classroom with the other students, pretended to examine the tadpole aquarium, and then walked straight to Miss Schmidt's desk in the front of the classroom. A majority of the students were in on the joke, so the room suddenly became quiet. This was such an unusual occurrence that Miss Schmidt looked up quickly, saw me standing in front of the desk, and said, "Yes, Steven?" At that point, my nerve rapidly began to desert me and I quavered, "Miss Schmidt, the tadpoles are all dead."

After a suitable pause to allow suspense to build, my plan was then to proclaim, "April Fool's!" But without skipping a beat, Miss Schmidt smoothly replied, "You may have five hours detention to clean the aquarium and set up the experiment again." I was stunned. The whole class was stunned. The joke had utterly backfired and I was to be significantly chastised. "But Miss Schmidt," I stammered, "it's April Fool's day. I was only joking." Whereupon just as quietly and firmly as her first pronouncement, she said, "So was I. April Fool's." And that was the one and only time unrestrained laughter was heard in the classroom of Miss Claudia Schmidt.

Why all these details about a seventh grade science teacher? How did all this influence my choice of a career in veterinary medicine? This austere disciplinarian had a rare love for the beauty of the natural world, a love she proceeded to communicate to her unruly and noisy students. Imagine, if you can, a group of fifteen students speaking in whispers and tiptoeing through a natural park within easy walking distance of the school—at seven a.m. before the start of classes. We stood in silence for minutes at a time listening to bird songs, catching brief glimpses of robins, cardinals, and blue jays. We were on a bird walk, learning to identify the various species living in the park, along with lessons of conservation, ecology, and botany. This was in the 1950s—long before conservation and ecology were the popular causes they are today.

From Miss Schmidt's seventh-grade bird walks, I became a lifelong devotee of bird watching. Even today, I rarely go anywhere without my bird books, binoculars, and life list of the birds I have identified. It was a natural consequence as I became involved in my chosen profession, and as many species of tropical birds became popular companion animals, that the diagnosis and treatment of these fascinating creatures assumed an ever-larger part of my professional practice.

Up to this time, I believed I wanted to be a veterinarian. I was attracted to animals and to the principles of medicine about which I was reading. But I had had little interaction with veterinarians except Dr. Donald Snow, our family veterinarian who tended to Duke's periodic health concerns in a matter-of-fact and kindly fashion. Dr. Snow heard constantly (as I do now) from young people about how much they love animals and want to be veterinarians when they grow up. Unfortunately, many veterinarians become cynical when we hear these declarations week after week. Thus, I received no particular encouragement from Dr. Snow in my expressed desire for a career in veterinary medicine. It falls to someone who wants such a career to pursue it, and to do so unwaveringly. In my case, I had a great deal of pursuing to do.

The final influence that solidified my determination for a career in veterinary medicine was a circus clown with a toothache. In the 1950s, Ringling Brothers Barnum and Bailey Circus was still touring smaller cities, including Springfield, Massachusetts. So it was, one evening in the spring of the mid-1950s when I was thirteen or fourteen years old, that our telephone rang and my father answered. After a few minutes of conversation, which included a surprised greeting of the caller by my father, I heard, "I'll meet you at my office in a few minutes." Dental emergencies were relatively rare, and those occasions when my father had to go back to his office after a long day were usually accompanied by mutterings about the distressed caller. This time, however, he went off to his office with apparent enthusiasm.

The call had come from a dental school classmate whom he had not seen in many years—and who was now the circus dentist. The chief clown, Felix Adler, had a terrible toothache that required equipment and materials he did not carry. My father not only opened his office and made all his equipment available, he also helped with the procedure, which relieved this important circus performer of his pain. In gratitude, Mr. Adler asked my father if there was anything he could do to express his thanks. My father replied, "Nothing for me, but I have a son who would love a pass to the circus." Mr. Adler immediately wrote out a lifetime pass in my name to Ringling Brothers Barnum and Bailey Circus.

What a thrill for me to receive this treasure from my father! I was not so thrilled about watching the circus performance as I was to meet a hero of mine, Dr. J.Y. Henderson—circus veterinarian and author of Circus Doctor, the first book written for the public about veterinary medicine in non-domestic species. Dr. Henderson was not only a pioneer in this field, but an enthralling author. I had read and reread his book several times (and continued to do so over the next several years). Dr. Henderson wrote of the diagnosis and treatment of health problems in lions, tigers, leopards, elephants, snakes, and other species about which little was known at that time. By applying the same principles he had learned and used in his previous practice with domestic species, especially horses, Dr. Henderson had made great progress understanding and treating the diseases and problems he was encountering with the circus collection. Circus Doctor played a pivotal role in the direction my career was to take.

This was the veterinarian with whom I was to spend two exciting days at the Ringling Brothers Circus—a time I will never forget. By his example, this man served as a role model for me in my continuing belief that veterinarians have an obligation to use their broad-ranging education to relieve disease and suffering throughout the animal kingdom, not just in the species with which they are most familiar. I have always felt that we veterinarians must take care lest we become specialists who know more and more about less and less—until we know everything about nothing.

chapter two

The Struggle to Open the Door

The die was cast. What I had been saying since age seven would come to pass. I would graduate from high school, attend and graduate from a college that offered pre-veterinary curriculum, and begin formal training in my chosen profession. It all seemed so logical, so straightforward, and attainable. I paid no attention to my parents who struggled to comprehend this family aberration; to my uncle, a maxillofacial surgeon, who asked, "Don't you want to be a real doctor?"; or to the results of my high school aptitude tests, which indicated my talents lay in a different direction. Despite the gloomy forecast from a college entrance counselor, I was accepted into the College of Arts and Sciences at Cornell University. That same campus in Ithaca, New York was the home of the New York State College of Veterinary Medicine, the closest veterinary college to my home state of Massachusetts.

My next four years were spent in what should have been ideal preparation for a career in veterinary medicine. All I had to do was to take and demonstrate ability in the pre-veterinary courses, mainly in the chemical and biological sciences, required for entrance to a college of veterinary medicine. The veterinary school at Cornell also required "farm practice" credits: two summers performing all aspects of practical farm work. Students were required to keep a detailed diary and pass an examination, both written and practical, upon completion. The assumption was that one could not possibly be a serious candidate for a career in veterinary medicine without the ability to take a milking machine apart and put it back together, or back a manure-spreader into a barn—two actual requirements for entry into the New York State College of Veterinary Medicine.

I successfully completed the farm practice requirements and passed the appropriate examination. I wish I could say the same about my endless chemistry, zoology, and genetics courses. What could these subjects possibly have to do with becoming a veterinary practitioner? I asked myself this question repeatedly. Were these courses a true measure of my ability to diagnose and treat the diseases of domestic and wild animals? If I couldn't calculate how many moles of solute were contained in a given chemical compound under conditions of standard temperature and pressure, or remember exactly to which subphylum the duckbilled platypus belonged, would I really be doomed to failure as a doctor of veterinary medicine?

Of much more practical value was the experience I received in canine behavior while living in a small fraternity house on the Cornell campus. Many years before my attendance at Cornell University, an extremely wealthy but rather eccentric elderly woman had left $1 million to the University, with the stipulation that dogs must be permitted in any and all buildings at the school, including the libraries and classrooms. Many fraternities are on the Cornell campus, and every one of them had at least one dog as a mascot. Some had several—and of course they tended to be the larger breeds—that roamed free over the picturesque campus. Dogs could be seen sunning themselves on the steps of the main library, attending various academic lectures, and even passing critical judgment on the quality of the food in the student cafeterias.

In my second year, our fraternity purchased a black German shepherd puppy whom we named Buddy. Because I was a pre-veterinary student and was supposed to know something about animals, the job of bringing up Buddy was delegated to me. Ordinarily this would not have been too much of a problem; however, there were twenty other members of the fraternity who often had different ideas about the way Buddy should behave and about how he should be trained. This sometimes led to much excitement.

As a puppy, Buddy was quite rambunctious and played rather roughly—a trait unfortunately encouraged by some of the fraternity members. What they failed to realize was that what was merely amusing puppy play would not be at all amusing when this puppy grew up to be a large, powerful dog. It wasn't quite fair to Buddy, I thought, to punish him for something others encouraged. However, something had to be done about the way Buddy used his (by now, quite large, strong) teeth during play.

One evening while Buddy and I were having a play/training session, he leaped up and bit my nose, missing my eye by not very much. Without thinking, I immediately turned and bit Buddy right on his cheek. I bit him hard enough so he let out a loud yelp and ran to the corner of the room. Although I have never heard this technique recommended by any dog trainer, and although I do not recommend that owners bite their dogs, I must report that Buddy never again used his teeth around human faces. In fact, Buddy always woke me up in the morning by nuzzling my face; after my little lesson, the minute my eyes opened Buddy quickly turned his face away from mine. I will leave to the judgment of other, more knowledgeable dog behaviorists and trainers as to whether I inflicted a cruel and unusual punishment on Buddy, but the results speak for themselves.

In general, canine activities on the Cornell campus were a far cry from responsible pet ownership; this often caused considerable problems, especially for the faculty. Once during one of my most crucial examinations, unbeknown to me, another fraternity member brought Buddy to the examination room. The professor giving the exam evidently was not as familiar with Cornell canine privileges as Buddy was, because he walked up to Buddy, who by this time was approaching 110 pounds, took him by the collar and started to evict him from the room. Buddy took extreme exception to this treatment. Engrossed in taking this difficult test, I was jolted out of my concentration by hearing a loud snarl and a terrified yell from the professor. Buddy had lunged at the man, backed him into a corner not far from my seat, and was advancing on him with the obvious intent of administering a severe reproof for the professor's outrageous ejection.

Horrified, I jumped out of my chair, took Buddy by the collar—making very sure he knew who I was—and hustled him out of the room. Using my belt as a leash, I handed the dog to a passing fraternity brother, told him what had happened, and said, "For god's sake, get him back to the house and lock him in a room till I get back." At least ten minutes had gone by, so I thought it was probably a waste of time to go back to the test room. I fully expected the professor to throw me out and fail me for the semester. Also, I would never be able to finish the exam in the remaining time allowed.

However, when I got back to the room to collect my things, the professor grabbed my hand and shook it frantically, thanking me for saving him from a savage mauling. He urged me back to my seat and promised me extra time to finish the test. I can't say with any certainty what influence Buddy had on my examination results, but I received a far higher grade than I expected, and passed the course with flying colors. Thank you, Buddy!

I don't mean to imply that my other pre-veterinary courses at Cornell lacked excitement or drama. One late evening I found myself in the genetics laboratory working on the crucial project of demonstrating the principles of genetics taught in our class lectures by breeding the Drosophila strain of fruit fly— whose physical characteristics were a humped back and white eyes (normal fruit flies have a straight back and reddish eyes). A high percentage of my grade in the genetics course depended on my success as a breeder of freak fruit flies. If I could not successfully and reliably breed fruit flies with these abnormal characteristics, and explain my method of doing so in proper genetic terms, I would definitely fail the course.

For readers not familiar with fruit flies: first, count your blessings, and second, please know that these creatures are one-tenth the size of the common housefly. They are quick and acrobatic fliers and are not easily caught (alive, at least). One has to use a microscope to examine their eyes and the shape of their back—provided, of course, you can persuade them to hold still long enough. Our method was to use ether, which rapidly put the flies to sleep for a detailed examination of the critical characteristics.

A few problems arose with this method, however. Because I needed these flies to breed after my examination and selection of the appropriate individuals, I had to use extreme caution not to give them too much ether, lest I create an anesthetic accident. Many evenings in that laboratory, I did have to restrain myself from having such an "accident."

To examine the little creatures, I had to get my microscope—and my nose—quite close to the etherized flies. This position was highly conducive to my becoming anesthetized in the process; it definitely impaired my powers of observation! Could a non-humpbacked or non-white-eyed fly have possibly gotten into my precious breeding stock? If so, it could invalidate my entire project—a sure sign I might well be an undesirable candidate for admission to a college of veterinary medicine.

Another problem associated with the project was that the fruit flies did not seem to understand what was expected of them; they made determined and often successful attempts to escape into the laboratory room. When this happened, I then had a choice: either I could let the little dears go free and populate the laboratory with offspring of whatever eye color and back shape they pleased, or I could attempt to recapture the escapees with a net, an endeavor that taxed every bit of athleticism I possessed. If video cameras had been readily at hand, someone could have produced a full-length comedy on life in a genetics laboratory. It would have needed to be a silent feature, however, for reasons not hard to imagine.

These examples notwithstanding, some true bright spots in my academic career came at Cornell University. Not all was drudgery in the pursuit of scientific excellence. My physics course is a good illustration. Because physics involved considerable mathematics, and clearly had nothing to do with animals,

I was apprehensive about the course. When the class average score on the first examination was 33 percent, I became even more worried about my chances of passing future examinations. Physics became one of the few courses for which I studied diligently. In the end, I received a numerical grade of 88 percent. I mention this because it was probably the highest grade I received in any of my courses during my four years at Cornell University, and it should have revealed that I was not entirely lacking in scientific ability. The problem was that my other science course grades did not reflect the same caliber of aptitude. For the most part, my academic record in the science courses was mediocre at best.

In fact, I committed what was, in that era, a cardinal sin. I did not elect a science field as my major area of academic concentration. Instead, I chose comparative dramatic literature as my major. Today, a veterinary college admissions committee would look upon that choice with interest, if not actual approval. Applicants to colleges of human medicine who majored in such subjects as philosophy, political science, or even English literature were judged to have broad interests that in the end would contribute positively to their medical careers. However, in the early '60s, skills such as backing a manure spreader and assembling a milking machine prevailed as prerequisites for veterinary college—and one ought to be at least competent in the basic sciences of chemistry, zoology, and physics.

Competition for spots in veterinary medicine programs was intense, and the colleges of veterinary medicine were not interested in admitting students who were unable to complete the course of study. One could gain acceptance to a college of human medicine more easily! At the time, it was the strong conviction of the colleges of veterinary medicine that your undergraduate record in the sciences was a good indicator of your ability to assimilate the large amount of material to be mastered in the four years of veterinary school.

In the early- to mid-'60s, seventeen schools in the United States and two in Canada offered a curriculum in veterinary medicine. All the schools in the U.S. were financially subsidized by the states where they were located. This meant admission preference was given to in-state applicants. What about students from states without colleges of veterinary medicine? Some states near those with veterinary schools made agreements to subsidize their students, who, in turn, were given some extra consideration. Third in priority were students from states with neither colleges of veterinary medicine nor regional agreements with states that did have veterinary colleges. Such was the situation with the Commonwealth of Massachusetts—of which I was an official resident.

If you combine a mediocre academic record in the sciences, an unconventional major field of study, residence in a state with neither veterinary college nor regional agreement with a state with a veterinary school, and at least twenty applicants for every available place in a class, you end up with an unattractive application—precisely what I was told by those schools to which I applied, including my undergraduate alma mater, Cornell University. Not one of the several schools so much as asked me to appear for a personal interview. A second application following a semester of postgraduate science courses at the University of Massachusetts likewise failed to convince any schools that I had reformed and deserved a chance.

Now began my true pursuit of a career in veterinary medicine—a journey of five years, marked by attempts to redeem my undesirable showing at Cornell and repeated rejections from numerous veterinary schools across the country. I took a three-and-a-half-year interlude with the U.S. Coast Guard. Most of that time I spent in Ketchikan, Alaska, cruising the magnificent, unspoiled, wild waters of Southeast Alaska on a 180-foot buoy tender—the U.S. Coast Guard cutter Balsam. This was, in itself, a great adventure; if ever I had been tempted to give up the idea of becoming a veterinarian, Alaska and its way of life presented a strong siren call.

Even in Alaska I maintained contact with veterinary medicine. Ketchikan, the fourth largest city in the state (population 7,000) had no veterinarian. The closest one was in Juneau, about 150 miles north as the crow (or Alaska Coastal Airlines) flies. Dr. Cliff Lobaugh came to Ketchikan once a month on the Alaska Marine ferry system; no roads connected any communities in Southeast Alaska so transportation was either via small airplanes that could land on water, or via boat.

Whenever Dr. Lobaugh arrived, he arranged a storeroom in one of the local supermarkets for his examination and operating room. If my ship was in port, I would assist him. Even as naive as I was about the practice of veterinary medicine, it seemed primitive to me that we should be performing ovariohysterectomies (otherwise known as "spay" surgeries) using a piece of covered plywood as an operating table. However Dr. Lobaugh seemed to be a skillful surgeon even under such conditions, and his results were successful. For anesthesia, he used the short-acting thiobarbiturate sodium pentothal—at that time a big step forward from the older, long-acting pentobarbital. Patients awoke quickly, but because modern pain medications were years in the future, many patients awoke in discomfort. They often "told" us about it for some time following surgery. Dr. Lobaugh and I stayed with these patients until we were sure it was safe to discharge them to their owners that evening. The ferry to Juneau was not until the next day, and Dr. Lobaugh was in the habit of simply spreading his sleeping bag on the floor of the storeroom to spend the night. As he explained, a night in an Alaskan hotel would pretty much wipe out any profit he might make from his visit. After my first experience helping Dr. Lobaugh with one of his storeroom surgeries, I invited him to stay with my wife and me at our place in town.

I well remember the first night he came to our tiny one-bedroom apartment. It was ten o'clock at night, and my wife Connie was sound asleep. I noticed Cliff Lobaugh tiptoeing around the living room as we pulled out the studio couch. He was speaking almost in whispers. In a normal voice, I asked him why he was whispering. He answered, "I don't want to wake up your wife." Now during my Alaska sojourn, I had developed a passion for Alaska king crab. Sensing an opportunity to enjoy this treat, I made the following wager with Dr. Lobaugh. I would stand at the foot of the bed and shout "Fire!" If my wife so much as twitched a toe, I would lose the bet. If she didn't move, I would win. We wagered a king crab dinner. I gently uncovered Connie's toes to prove to Cliff she would not awaken, shouted at the top of my lungs, and … the result? Fresh king crab never tasted better.

As idyllic as our life in Alaska was, it came time to choose whether to stay there or transfer my final year on Coast Guard active duty to somewhere I could improve my academic record, reapply to veterinary colleges, and have a better chance of acceptance. In the autumn of 1965, after two-and-a-half adventurous years as a deck watch officer on the Balsam, my wife and I were transferred to U.S. Coast Guard headquarters for the Great Lakes area Search and Rescue division in Cleveland, Ohio. Cleveland's prestigious medical school at Western Reserve University (now Case-Western) was where I could take some advanced science/medical courses that would prove, once and for all, whether I had what it took to complete the course of study in veterinary medicine. The plan was all well and good, but can you imagine the shock we felt, coming from the pristine wilderness of Alaska, as we drove by the horribly polluted water of Lake Erie and rolled up our car windows because of the stench.

I had one final year on active duty in the Coast Guard, yet I was still determined to make a career in veterinary medicine my reality. I was advised that as a member of the U.S. military, my Massachusetts residency—a disadvantage to me on my previous two applications—would be waived on all applications. I would now be considered a resident of the entire country. I was also three years older and had been in charge of various aspects of a U.S. military unit. These things ought to count for something, I reasoned. Not far from Cleveland was the Ohio State College of Veterinary Medicine in Columbus. I decided to talk to the dean of the school and get accurate and authoritative guidance on the quickest, surest way to be accepted. I would follow the dean's advice and surely be on my way.

I drove to Columbus, arriving early so I could walk around the campus and imagine what it would be like to be one of the chosen few—a member of a respected profession who would devote the rest of my life to relieving the suffering of animals. I would be a colleague (what a wonderful term) of my early hero, Dr. J.Y. Henderson—the "circus doctor." It was thrilling to think of that dream becoming a possibility.

I was ushered into the office of Dean Krill, who seemed interested, friendly, and supportive of my career objectives. I had brought transcripts of my academic records at Cornell and the University of Massachusetts. When he had listened to my personal history (written resumes were not in vogue at that time) and looked at my transcripts, his comment was, "Frankly, your academic record needs improvement. You are more mature now than when you graduated. You can apply for admission this year, but if I were you, I would take some good, tough science courses and bolster your record. Then you will have a better chance for admission." I was not disappointed by these comments; I had expected them. I had come to Cleveland ready to take "good, tough science courses," and when I was discharged from active duty next year that is exactly what I intended to do. Just in case, I did apply to Ohio State as well as Cornell, but was not accepted nor granted an interview—as Dean Krill had predicted. This made failed attempt number three in my struggle to be accepted to a veterinary program.

As soon as I was discharged from active Coast Guard duty early in 1966, I began taking medical school level courses at Western Reserve University: histology, embryology, and comparative anatomy. I began work in the germ-free research laboratory at the medical school working for veterinarian Dr. Aaron Leash, a graduate of Michigan State University College of Veterinary Medicine. In theory, if my work impressed him, I could count on a letter of recommendation—a positive addition to my application. Both the work and the courses went smoothly, and although I didn't set the world on fire with scholarship, my grades were considerably better than during my undergraduate days at Cornell.

I looked forward to a favorable outcome for my next round of applications.

One important addition to our family occurred near the end of our first year in Cleveland: My wife, who had not grown up with dogs, yielded—somewhat reluctantly—to my desire for a canine companion. First, we had to agree upon a breed. I wanted a Doberman pincher, a breed that had fascinated me for many years. Their alert athleticism and trim, clean appearance was aesthetically appealing as was their obvious trainability. On the other hand, my wife was fearful of their reputation as vicious and aggressive "killers"—a ridiculous picture spurred on by periodic sensational journalism. They just didn't look cuddly, my wife pointed out. Visitors to our house might be intimidated. Reluctantly, I had to admit she was right. So we looked in the American Kennel Club book, which listed some 124 recognized breeds, and discussed the advantages and disadvantages of all possible candidates.

Out of the 124 breeds listed, my wife and I could agree on only one: the German shorthaired pointer. They had the long floppy ears that seemed to be prerequisite for cute and cuddly, and they were both outdoorsy and companion house dogs. With that tentative agreement, I began contacting breeders in the area. In the interim my wife had to make a trip back to see her parents in Springfield, Massachusetts. While she was gone, a breeder nearby happened to have a small litter of three puppies about eight weeks of age—just right for a new home. When I met my wife at the airport in Cleveland a few days later I said, "We have a small detour to make on the way home." We went to see the puppies, and I said to Connie, "Pick any puppy you love." Somewhat dazed by the rapidity of events, she picked one of the male pups. We named him "Kin" after one of the dog characters in Albert Payson Terhune's collie stories (all of which I read and reread as a child). Although we were living in a suburban community, Connie was a full-time teacher, and I was taking classes at Western Reserve University, we still found time to take daily walks and weekend romps in local woodlands with Kin. He became one of the delights of our life in Cleveland, and he learned basic obedience with bewildering speed and ease. This meant we could take him with us almost everywhere we went. In fact, shortly after we got Kin, my wife attended a wedding in Delaware. I drove twelve hours from Cleveland to meet her with little Kin curled up beside me on the seat of our Volkswagen bug. All he needed was a few extra stops: It was much easier than traveling with a child.

As a veterinarian, all too often I have people ask me to put their pets to sleep or help them find new homes for their companions because they are moving and can't take their pets with them. Some of these animals have been in the family for many years. Inwardly, I was always greatly angered when confronted with this situation. Do people think pets are only for their convenience? And that they can be cast aside when there are problems? I wondered. In fact, in almost every case, I have found that if an owner takes the time and trouble, they need not abandon these family members.

Several months after we got Kin, we moved from the west side of Cleveland to a suburb on the opposite side of the city called Shaker Heights, to be close to Connie's teaching position in that community. The community was in a quiet, attractive area with many trees and parks. Several older two-family homes were owned by people who lived in one half and rented out the other. We left Kin in the car and went to look at one of these homes in a lovely neighborhood. We fell in love with the house and the area. Connie and I quickly decided we wanted to live in that house for however long we remained in Cleveland. However, there was one problem: The advertisement in the newspaper had specified "no pets."

I approached the homeowner who had shown us the house and said, "Now I would like you to meet another member of our family." I went to the car, put young Kin on his leash, and proceeded to command him through his obedience routine: heel, sit, down, stay, and come. As I did, I watched the landlady out of the corner of my eye. When I first took Kin out of the car I saw her head shake "no, no, no." But as I continued to demonstrate Kin's good manners and training and the care we were obviously taking with him, the head-shaking stopped. I walked over to the landlady and told her, "I am prepared to write out a check right now for whatever amount you specify as a damage deposit, although I'm confident that there will be no damage, because Kin is never alone for more than three or four hours." Apparently, no one had ever approached her in that manner before. She hesitated for a short while and asked us a few questions about our daily routine, but in the end, she agreed to allow us to live in her house with a written stipulation that we would be required to leave if Kin was noisy or destructive. This is just one example of how to approach a problem often faced by pet owners who must move and who do not own their own homes. It was utterly unthinkable that we give up Kin, and that must be the initial attitude of any owner who deals with this situation. As we will see, there are other strategies as well.

In that lovely old home in Shaker Heights, there was a fireplace in the living room. The owner assured us it was a working fireplace, so we bought a small

S T E V E N   B .   M E T Z ,   D . V . M .

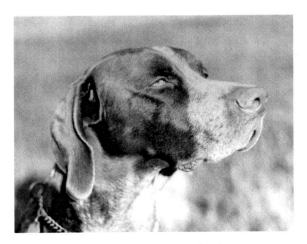

Kin was the Metz family's German shorthair pointer.

supply of firewood. One chilly evening we built a fire and enjoyed a leisurely visit with some friends. We kept the fire going for several hours before letting it burn out. Connie and I had our bedroom at the opposite end of the house from the fireplace. Kin slept in the bedroom with us—as all our dogs have since. Around four a.m. the next morning, Kin awakened us with loud and insistent barking. He hardly ever barked, so we woke up immediately and noticed the air in the bedroom seemed smoky. I got up to investigate and heard a loud banging on the front door. Throwing on a bathrobe, I ran to the door and started to choke—the living room was full of smoke. I opened the door just as some firemen were preparing to break it down. They shouted that the third floor above us was in flames and we had to get out right now. Forget any belongings, they yelled, just get out!

Fortunately, the fire was in the early stages, and the fire department was able to bring it under control with minimal damage to the floors below. The cause was insufficient insulation and improper construction of the old fireplace. It had been constructed as a gas fireplace and had not been used for many years. The firemen might have rescued us even if Kin had not awakened us, but it is undeniable that he understood something was terribly wrong and we needed to pay attention. Find another home for Kin when we moved again? Not likely!

It was now time to make my fourth application for admission to veterinary school, and I scheduled an appointment with the dean of the veterinary school at Michigan State University in East Lansing, an almost twelve-hour drive from Cleveland in those years. The day I went, there happened to be a snow-storm, and I had to drive almost twelve hours overnight to reach East Lansing. I remember being somewhat on edge from the hazardous drive when I was ushered into the office of Dean W. W. Armistead. To this day, forty-six years later, I remember what followed. Without much preliminary conversation, Dean Armistead said, "Ah, Mr. Metz. I see you are from Massachusetts. We here at Michigan State are sick and tired of taking care of Massachusetts castoffs. Frankly, I don't think you have a hope in hell of getting into Michigan State College of Veterinary Medicine. Good day, Mr. Metz." I was stunned. If ever there was an outright repudiation of my hopes for becoming a veterinarian, that five-minute "interview" was it. There was not much reply to be made, so I excused myself and drove ten-and-a-half hours back to Cleveland—through the same storm. I did not apply to Michigan State College of Veterinary Medicine, despite a good recommendation from Dr. Leash.

This was an unexpectedly poor beginning to my fourth attempt at acceptance. However, I was making some progress: Cornell University finally granted me an interview. Perhaps I could convince them after four applications that I was serious about veterinary medicine, that I had the determination and the mental capacity to do well in the curriculum, and that I deserved a chance to prove myself. So with great hope (after all, this was my alma mater), I drove to Ithaca, New York for my first interview with an admissions committee. I also planned to get advice from Dr. William I. Myers, the grandfather of my college roommate, with whom I had remained and still remain very close since graduation. This was no ordinary grandfather. He had been the dean of the Cornell University College of Agriculture for many years. His prestige was formidable, even though he was now retired. If I could make a good impression on him, I could at least get the best possible advice on appealing to the admissions committee, if not an outright recommendation or intervention on my behalf. But I was in for more plain talk. After receiving me cordially this wonderful gentleman cut right to the heart of the matter: "Well, Steven, you say you want to be a veterinarian. How do you explain your lousy record in the sciences?"

I have had many a chuckle over this episode in recent years, but at the time, I was reduced to stammering excuses that sounded lame, even to me. Yes, I had recently done better, and I was older and more mature, but I still had considerable explaining to do about my undergraduate record at this very school where the next day I would face a committee dedicated to weeding out would-be veterinary students from the real article.

I cannot recall the exact composition of the admissions committee, but I do recall that several were members of the faculty of the veterinary college. They were, quite naturally, interested in hearing an explanation of my previous shortcomings as a student of the basic sciences—the foundation for the future curriculum to which I aspired. Dr. Francis Fox, professor of large animal medicine, delivered the final "nail in the coffin" when he demanded, "Mr. Metz, I see you majored in literature. What are you going to do, read Shakespeare to the cows?" My reply was that such studies would equip me to communicate with owners of my patients, be they cows, pigs, or—heaven forbid—dogs and cats. I say "heaven forbid" because at that time in veterinary medicine, companion animal veterinarians—or "small animal" veterinarians—were viewed as catering to a luxury. The real veterinarian devoted himself (at that time, it was an overwhelmingly male-dominated profession) to food animal medicine: "large animals" only.

Alas, neither my renewed academic efforts at Western Reserve University medical school nor my theories on client communication impressed the members of this admissions committee, and for the fourth time my application was rejected. The University of California at Davis, Colorado State University, and Washington State University informed me they would not accept applications from out-of-state students from states without regional agreements. Kansas State University required a poultry husbandry course—required by no other veterinary college—which I most certainly did not have. My options were dwindling. But I still had an opportunity, I thought, at Ohio State. I had followed the advice of Dean Krill and taken courses in a medical school. My grades were above average in these upper level courses. That ought to count for something!

Back I went to the affable Dean Krill at Ohio State College of Veterinary Medicine with preliminary transcripts of the courses I had taken at Western Reserve University. He read the transcripts, and I respectfully reminded him of our conversation the previous year. Dean Krill sat behind his desk in a tilt-back chair. He said to me, "Frankly, my boy, this time I'm in your corner. Of course, I'm only one of three members of the final admissions committee but I'm definitely in your corner."

As I eagerly watched the mail, my hopes rested on Ohio State. I wasn't expecting word from them for at least several weeks, but rejections from other schools were coming in. Dean Krill, I hoped, really was "in my corner." In mid-spring, an envelope arrived at last. I opened it with a mixture of anticipation and dread. It was an outright rejection—and even earlier than the rejection I received when Dean Krill was not in my corner.

For the first time in the five years I had been trying to gain entry to veterinary medicine, I began to have serious doubts about the eventual outcome. To whom could I turn? What could I do to change those colleges' impressions— that I was unfit for a career in veterinary medicine? Perhaps, after all, I was unfit. All the voices around me were shouting for me to recognize the truth. Besides every veterinary school to which I had applied, my wife and my parents were gently calling on me to recognize that my talents lay elsewhere, and I should get on with my life.

The absolute low point, perhaps of my life to that point, came when I asked my professor of embryology at Western Reserve for a letter of recommendation for some additional applications. I had completed his embryology course with an above average grade and had worked particularly diligently on the material. I was bewildered when this professor told me that he could not, in good conscience, write a letter of recommendation for me. I was not accustomed to questioning the decisions of any of my professors, but in this case, I blurted out, "Sir, do you mind explaining why not?" Beyond all the rejections, the refusals, and the negative comments I had received to this point, this one really hit home, and left me numb with hurt.

"First," he said, "I don't believe you are medical or veterinary school material. I don't believe you can be accepted at any school. But if you were accepted, I don't think you could complete the course. If you did somehow manage to complete the course, you would finish at the bottom of your class." This was not some random academician or untutored third party or even a member of an admissions committee selecting a prospective student from a pool of applicants. This was a respected professor in whose classroom I had spent a semester of hard work. He truly was in a position to evaluate my academic potential.

This felt to me like the final judgment. I had no reserves left to cope with a pronouncement like this one. I went back to our home and sat staring out a window. I would have to quit. Determination and perseverance were one thing, futility was quite another. If this respected professor's evaluation was accurate, if this was actually the light in which I was viewed by admissions committees reviewing my credentials, there now seemed absolutely no hope, no reasonable expectation that any amount of work or other preparation would change any opinions.

In reading this tale, please think about the influence one person can have upon another's life—for better or for worse. When I was a high school student, the guidance counselor whose job it was to assist students with their academic career planning, told me that I would most likely not be accepted to Cornell University and should not bother to apply. That counselor was wrong. Likewise, with no room left for doubt, I was judged unfit by a respected professor to enter a profession that had been my lifelong hope. I have no doubt he was entirely sincere in his pronouncement, but he was wrong, too, as you will see.

Meanwhile, unbeknown to me, my older brother—Dr. Lawrence Metz, a neurologist in Springfield, Massachusetts—had been treating Dr. Ronald North, a veterinary practitioner, for some nerve damage in one arm and hand. My brother helped with the diagnosis of the problem and recommended a surgeon to help Dr. North. If the surgery was not performed, Dr. North would eventually lose the use of his hand and would not be able to continue practicing. Dr. North was apprehensive about surgery because it was a rather delicate procedure; if there were any problems, he might lose some or all of the use of his hand. Happily, the outcome was excellent, and Dr. North regained full use of his hand. He told my brother that he had saved his career, and that he would do anything to help my brother in any way. My brother told Dr. North about my struggle for acceptance into veterinary school. Dr. North was a graduate of the Ontario Veterinary College in Canada, the first and oldest veterinary college in North America. I had never applied to that particular school because when I requested admissions information, their admissions office let me know that they were not accepting applicants from the United States. But the entrance requirements for the Ontario Veterinary College had changed that very year. The province of Ontario's high schools had a grade thirteen. Until this year, the Ontario Veterinary College had required completion of grade thirteen plus one year of pre-veterinary science courses. This had just been changed to two years of pre-veterinary study. Because of this change—and for that year only—the Ontario Veterinary College was short of qualified applicants from their usual group of Ontario and other Canadian students. In addition, I had an aggressive and demanding advocate who was an alumnus: Dr. Ronald North. I am not sure to this day whether Dr. North used the telephone, personal visits, or both. I do know he forcibly argued that if the Ontario Veterinary College wanted the financial support of its American alumni, it had better admit one Steven Metz.

After filling out a routine application and submitting transcripts, I was accepted to the Ontario Veterinary College class of 1970. Everything happened so fast and was so unexpected that I went through the motions as if it were all a dream. Could it really be true? I was going to get my chance. I was going to be able to stop talking about being a veterinarian and do it. Now the doubts began. Could I do the work? I really had never studied in a concentrated, single-minded way. I owed it to Dr. North, the only person besides my family who had actually been in my corner, and I owed it to myself after all the years of hearing people tell me that I was unfit for the profession. I would vindicate Dr. North and prove all the "professionals" wrong. I would work as I had never worked at anything before.

chapter three

My Amazing Veterinary Education

The Ontario Veterinary College is located in Guelph, Ontario, Canada. When I was admitted, Guelph was a small city an hour west of Toronto with a population of 49,000. I had just had knee surgery and was on crutches just in time to be not much help in packing all our belongings. We knew absolutely no one in the Guelph area, and not much about crossing the Canadian border with a moving van. Several weeks in advance, I had called Canadian Customs and Immigration Services in Niagara Falls. I was told that as a student I was allowed to bring household goods, nothing complicated about it. An unwelcome surprise awaited us when we arrived at the border and were informed we could not bring household goods across the border without prior arrangements and an exact list and description of every item. Additionally, because we were going to be in Canada for four years, we would have to apply for landed immigrant status—meaning we would have to sign a declaration that we intended to give up our U.S. citizenship, and we would become Canadian citizens. When I protested that I had called in advance and was told nothing about these requirements, the customs officer growled, "They should have told you that."

We resolved the problem, believe it or not, by opening up enough cartons for inspection to convince the customs officer there really were that many books and phonograph records. The immigrations officer agreed to let us go to Guelph, but I was going to have to be interviewed by local immigrations officials within a few days of our arrival. Welcome to Canada!

It didn't matter; we were so deliriously happy for this chance that we'd jump through any hoops required. Thus we three arrived in Guelph with all our worldly goods, a rented van, a Volkswagen Bug, Kin, and a 65-cc Honda motorbike. Our first task was to find a house or apartment for the next four years. We quickly found out that Guelph landlords were not enthusiastic about students, even married ones, with dogs. We kept looking and soon found a little house eight miles away from Guelph. The landlords, Mr. and Mrs. Anton Schavo, professed to be dog breeders and enthusiasts. They said they were delighted to have Kin live in their house. The place was in Eden Mills—population 40, which I believe qualifies it as a hamlet.

It was a good thing that during our time in Alaska, I had a bush pilot friend fly Connie out to a Tlingit Indian fishing village named Klawock (Alaska enthusiasts: try to find that one on a map), which had about the same population—except the Tlingit village had two bars that were very lively at night. Eden Mills, Ontario, by contrast, had one general store and an on-again-off-again sawmill powered by a waterwheel and the tiny Eramosa River that ran through the center of town. The Eramosa widened out to a little pond because of the milldam. This pond and the river were fifty yards from our Eden Mills house.

Our new home was quite unlike any place Connie or I had ever experienced, and it was to provide us with some exciting moments. It was at the top of a small hill and had no driveway. Parking was no problem, however, because we were at the end of a dirt lane (100 yards from the general store), so we just drove to the end of the lane and stopped. The hill seemed extra steep when we had groceries or other things to carry into the house, especially in the winter. We devised ways to cope that made it fun. Just down the hill and across the lane was an English couple who owned a very large, very friendly, very slobbery Saint Bernard named Pandora. She was to give us some exciting moments. She and Kin became fast friends; we just had to wipe off the slobber after they finished playing.

In the few days before classes started, Connie and I tried to familiarize ourselves with our Eden Mills neighbors (quite few in number) and with the city of Guelph, the Ontario Veterinary College, and the Canadian Immigration Service. Step one was to introduce Kin to the neighbors. As well behaved as he was, I almost never allowed him off-leash. But fifty acres of pasture and woodlands served as our backyard, and it would be a pity if he could not have a good run and some activity appropriate to his breed while we lived in such a setting. So that residents in the vicinity would recognize him and know he had a concerned owner on the slim chance he ever became lost, I knocked on all the neighbors' doors and introduced Kin and myself. I politely but emphatically mentioned that Kin was a beloved member of our family, that he was never let out unaccompanied, but that if ever he were lost I would appreciate any help in recovering him. Most were surprised by my concern; after all, it was farm country, and there were no leash laws. They listened in the quietly reserved and polite Canadian way to which we would become accustomed over the next four years.

The city of Guelph seemed connected in large part to the Ontario Veterinary College and Ontario Agricultural College. The schools were on either side of the main highway running through the city. After negotiating the difficulties of working in a foreign country, as pointed out by the friendly Canadian immigrations officer, Connie promptly secured a position as French language teacher at the Guelph High School. The immigrations officer was puzzled by our reluctance to give up our U.S. citizenship. After all, he pointed out, our country was torn by race riots and other socially undesirable conditions. Why did we not jump at the chance to become Canadian citizens? Of course we were anxious not to offend a government official during the first days of what we hoped would be a four-year stay, so we had to be careful in answering his questions. Somehow we were able to satisfy him that there was hope we would eventually see the error of our ways and become Canadians. With all these vital concerns under control, at age twenty-seven—after four years of rejections plus three years in the U.S. Coast Guard—I began the studies that would lead to my lifelong career in veterinary medicine.

Sixty-five students gathered in the anatomy laboratory for our first class. About one-third of the students were from the United States because of the change in entrance requirements. Four Americans had transferred from a veterinary school in the Philippines where they had already completed their first year of study, but they would receive no credit for it because the Philippine school was not accredited by the American Veterinary Medical Association or the Canadian Veterinary Medical Association. Nevertheless, they had studied anatomy and other basic subjects and had a definite advantage over the rest of the class. Several students hailed from western Canada and had a mysterious rapport with one another from the outset. One student was from India, one from Nigeria, two were from the West Indies, and one was from Japan. All the foreign students except the Japanese man spoke excellent English and seemed to have no difficulty with written materials or lectures. Alas, the Japanese student could not manage, even when given oral examinations and extraordinary latitude by the college. He did not complete his first year.

The door to the laboratory room opened and a stocky man with extraordinarily bushy eyebrows and a long white lab coat walked in. "My name is J. H. Ballantyne of the Department of Anatomy. We here at the Ontario Veterinary College do not intend to turn a bunch of incompetents loose on an unsuspecting public. Get to work."

This was our welcome to the Ontario Veterinary College. We looked at each other and got to work learning the anatomy of the dog, horse, and cow (or ox as the anatomy text termed cattle). Our first year was also occupied mastering biochemistry, basic animal husbandry, physiology, embryology, histology, and introductory pathology. Some of us also received an introduction to the British system of education, namely that in most of our courses there would be only one examination—the "final"—at the end of the academic semester. There would be none of the academic handholding American students were accustomed to—that is, periodic quizzes and smaller examinations designed to warn a student who was not understanding the material. We were entirely responsible for learning the material presented to us. The faculty of the Ontario Veterinary College was a wonderful mixture of Australians, Europeans, Brits, Canadians, and Americans. This melding of medical and professional educations and philosophies resulted in a far more varied education than the one I would have received at a typical school in the United States—not necessarily better, but quite different.

I often awoke in the middle of the night during that first year feeling outright fear of failure. So many years of listening to people who were supposed to know what they were talking about tell me I was not "medical school material" or my "skills lay in another area." Could they be right? Well, except for anatomy, I faired pretty well. All of the class had difficulty with the sheer volume of material to be memorized. I had particular difficulty with anatomy because I was a poor sketcher, whereas some of my classmates could almost reproduce the textbook drawings of bones, muscles, joints, nerves, blood vessels, and their relationship to each other. Keeping his promise of not turning "incompetents loose on an unsuspecting public," Professor Ballantyne made sure his examinations were detailed, rigorous, and imaginative. In turn, some answers he received were also quite imaginative. Here is a typical test question: "The pointer indicates one of the mammary glands on a female dog. Name the exact structure." Not knowing the exact name required, one student answered, "George." Confirming his initial impression, Dr. Ballantyne made sure to let the entire class know that levity, which he equated with incompetence, was particularly unacceptable in the anatomy lab.

Another examination question involved a bone completely enclosed in an opaque bag. We were required to reach into the bag, feel the bone and identify it; name the species of animal to which it belonged, and indicate whether it came from the left or right side of the animal. At the end of the year, I had passed all my courses, but just squeaked by in anatomy.

To help pay for my education, I took a job at the Ontario Veterinary College's research farm where, among other programs, there was an ongoing study of hemophilia in a particular colony of 127 Walker hound dogs. My position was caretaker of these 127 dogs, and the job required twice daily cleaning of their individual quarters and twice daily feeding. Periodically these dogs had blood samples taken for studies on the bleeding disorder. As a beginning student I was not allowed to draw their blood, because they had a great tendency to bleed for long periods after any wound. They required someone with expert venipuncture technique—either a graduate veterinarian or the head technician on the farm, who had been there for over ten years. He was truly expert and I watched him as much as possible to learn the skill essential for any practicing veterinarian, namely to get a needle or catheter into a vein quickly and with minimum discomfort to the patient, whether it be a dog, cat, cow, or horse. (Drawing blood from birds and reptiles was far from my mind at that stage of my career.)

From this head technician, I had the first installment of a lesson on assuming things—a lesson I frequently recount to other veterinarians, technicians, and my clients. One day after work, this head technician came to me, "I know you're not yet a graduate veterinarian, but I'm sure you can help me with this. My dog at home seems to be constipated, and I thought an enema would help, do you?" I agreed (which in itself was improper to do) and gave him a small, prepackaged enema, such as anyone could purchase at a drugstore. I cautioned him to make sure to take the dog outside right after giving the enema.

Later that evening I got an angry call at home: "I know I should make allowances because you are not yet a veterinarian, but if you ever get to be one I hope you never do to someone else's pet what you've done to my dog. I gave her the enema that you okayed over an hour ago, and she hasn't stopped vomiting and drooling since!"

He had given the enema by mouth! Who would have believed it? Everyone knows where an enema is given, don't they? I had assumed a man of his experience would know. The mistake of assuming was mine alone and the lesson went into my subconscious notebook.

During the summer following my first year, I made the acquaintance of the local veterinarian in Guelph, Dr. Norman Hawkins, who operated a modest private small animal practice in the city, within a few miles of the prestigious Ontario Veterinary College's small animal clinic. In the coming four years while I was a student at OVC, a valuable part of my education was learning to deal with professional rivalries—which exist, I'm sure, in every profession, but never more fiercely than in medicine (human and otherwise). The fact that Dr. Hawkins could operate a successful veterinary practice so close to a college of Veterinary Medicine meant that more than a few pet owners were dissatisfied with the care that they or their pets received at the college. Thus, long before surveys and polls, I learned the importance of client relations—still the number one concern of all veterinary practice managers. I also learned about relations with one's professional colleagues—a skill and an obligation that, I am sorry to say, was and still is neglected in our veterinary education, and a difficult challenge throughout the medical professions.

The start of my second year was accompanied by considerable foreboding because everyone knew it was by far the most difficult academically. In crude terms, we would apply our backsides to a chair in the lecture hall from 8 a.m. to 5 p.m. with just a short break for lunch. We would be expected to assimilate a tremendous amount of theoretical material. In all my years as a student, I had never developed the kind of study habits that understanding this amount of material would demand. I would have to do something drastic to make sure I was successful in this difficult year. So I adopted this routine for the entire second year at the Ontario Veterinary College. I have never done anything like it before or since:

1. Finish classes at 5 p.m.

2. Immediately come home to our little house in Eden Mills and have an early supper

3. Select three subjects for the evening's attention and assemble all the materials needed for their study

4. Starting no later than 7 p.m., set an alarm clock for exactly one hour, and begin study on the first subject

5. When the alarm rings, immediately put the first subject down (even if in the middle of a paragraph and take a ten-minute break

6. Repeat the above routine with subjects two and three

7. At 10:30 p.m. put away all study material; take Kin out for a short walk around Eden Mills and go to bed

I repeated this routine for the entire academic year. I also developed one other study habit that provoked a reaction among my classmates. To make certain I understood the lecture material presented, I asked questions, many questions. I asked so many questions that the professors began to flinch when they saw my hand rise. My classmates began the "Metz Question Pool." Each day, the participants would bet on how many questions I would ask during the day's lectures. At the end of the day I would be the recipient of satisfied smiles from the winners, scowls from the losers, and frustrated frowns from just about everyone who wanted to get out of the lectures quickly.

Occasionally, my questions provided opportunity for general amusement, as happened when I questioned our professor of surgery, Dr. James Archibald—one of the most famous veterinary surgeons in North America at the time, and author of the first textbook on canine surgery. He was giving a lecture on following sterile, or "aseptic," procedures in the operating room. I raised my hand and blurted out, "Sir, is the anesthetist sterile?" He looked at me for a minute, allowing the suspense to build, then replied, "I've never questioned him about the subject, but next time we're out socially and he's had enough to drink, I'll try to find out for you." The whole class exploded with laughter, and I had a very red face.

All was not simply book learning, even at this early stage in our education. My classmate Wolf Zenker was, along with his wife, a breeder and show exhibitor of purebred Burmese cats and had twelve females in their home. I had almost no experience with cats, and certainly never lived with one, but these beautiful and personable, rich sable-brown Burmese cats with their outgoing personalities and expressive, often-used voices were another matter. I fell in love and wanted to add one to our family. My long-suffering wife had serious doubts about more animals in general, and cats in particular. I prevailed on my classmate and Connie to have Penny, a young female Burmese kitten, come stay with us as a trial.

The final decision was made considerably easier after the Zenkers received a male Burmese cat from a cattery in Texas for breeding purposes. A few days after the arrival of this Texas cat, several and then all of the cats began to sneeze and express ocular and nasal discharge. This progressed to a loss of appetite due to the stuffy noses, sore throats and tongues; we could actually see ulcers in the mouths of some of these poor, sick cats. There was no mystery about the diagnosis: upper respiratory infections caused by several different viruses, the two most dangerous of which were rhinotracheitis virus and calicivirus. The Texas cat had obviously been a carrier, and the Zenker cats were susceptible.

This was well before any vaccine had been developed to protect cats from these virulent, dangerous viruses. Also, antibiotics do not affect viruses living inside the body's cells. In other words, no specific treatment existed for these terribly sick cats. Yet, we were at the Ontario Veterinary College, the source and repository of all the latest knowledge and techniques for treating illnesses of all sorts. Surely, some of our professors could explain what must be done to treat and save the cats?

Alas, here was my first experience with helplessness. While my "borrowed" kitten, Penny, was happy and healthy at my Eden Mills home, my classmate and I watched while, one after another, his formerly beautiful, sleek, vibrantly alive cats died. They died no matter what we did, no matter what medications we gave; they died no matter that we gave each cat electrolyte fluid injections several times a day, and no matter that in our desperation we finally started feeding the cats by nasogastric tubes—the same method used with people who cannot eat.

Every one of those poor cats died, in spite of all the devoted nursing care Wolf Zenker, his wife, and I could give them, and in spite of advice from our professors. Years later, an effective vaccine was developed to protect cats from these deadly viruses. For a practitioner who could now prevent such heart-breaking illnesses and deaths, the vaccine was a godsend. Having seen pets suffer and die, not only from feline upper respiratory disease, but from many other diseases (canine distemper and parvovirus, to list only two of the deadliest viruses affecting our pets), I have little patience for people who blame vaccines for all sorts of health problems.

Many veterinarians today are trying to reduce the number and frequency of the vaccines given to pets. This approach certainly has some merit, but many younger practitioners have never seen cases of the devastating diseases some of we earlier graduates have had to face. I might be accused of resisting change, but I hope never again to witness anything like the illness and death of those twelve beautiful animals. Vaccines, whatever their drawbacks, can and do prevent needless deaths.

Despite the fact that our kitten Penny was the only remaining cat of the Zenkers' breeding, they gave her to us—partly as thanks for the day and night nursing we had done trying to save the group. Our family was expanded by one lovely, personable Burmese cat, who had narrowly escaped death because of our tryout. Penny lived with us for fourteen wonderful years. Her little pawprint, along with Kin's, remain in the concrete walk in the entrance to my Shelburne Veterinary Hospital.

As our second year at OVC drew to a close, we all looked forward to the beginning of clinical work with actual sick patients. Our book learning often seemed so unconnected with the real world of veterinary medicine that we

Steven B. Metz, d.v.m.

were quite impatient to get to the heart of our education. As for me, the strict study discipline paid off. I finished the year in the top ten of my class, the first time I had ever been in such a position.

I spent the summer working for Dr. Norm Hawkins at the Guelph Animal Hospital, learning the difference between the "ivory tower" academic approach we were taught at the college and the real world of private veterinary practice. Perhaps Dr. Hawkins was amused and attracted by my sheer enthusiasm and naiveté, and I suspect he took as much pleasure in exposing me to reality as I did in telling him about all the latest new approaches to problems—with which he'd been dealing simply and efficiently for years.

A good example of the clash between reality and academia was found in the most commonly performed canine and feline surgery: the ovariohysterectomy, or "spay" surgery, in which both ovaries and the uterus are removed. Several good reasons support performing this surgery, chief among them population control. Unrestrained reproduction in our dog and cat population has resulted in the necessity for humane societies and animal shelters in most communities all across the United States and Canada. Their mission is to find homes for the stray and unwanted residents or destroy them humanely (although some financially well-endowed shelters have "no-kill" policies, meaning they care for pets as long as they live). If surgical sterilization—the ovariohysterectomy and neutering surgeries—were practiced scrupulously by all pet owners, there would be no need for these shelters or for euthanizing the thousands upon thousands of unwanted dogs and cats that are a result of careless owners who allow indiscriminate breeding.

I could fill a chapter with stories from owners, "morning-after" stories I call them, about how they just let their female out the back door for five minutes, or they thought the fence around the back yard was high enough, or they tied their dog out on the lawn but the rope or collar broke. None of them ever dreamed such a thing could happen so fast. Of course, they thought, there was no reason to worry about finding homes for the puppies or kittens—the neighbor or the coworker at the office had said they wanted one. Unfortunately, all too often the friend or neighbor's response to an imminent litter is, "You mean now?"

Another purely medical reason for the ovariohysterectomy surgery is the prevention of breast cancer—one of the most common cancers in female dogs and cats, and almost completely preventable if pets have this common surgery before their reproductive organs mature. Spaying also will prevent uterine infection, common among females who neither have the surgery nor are bred. This condition, known as pyometra, usually requires an ovariohysterectomy as soon as possible—except the surgery is being done on a sick patient, turning a routine procedure into a tricky and often hazardous one. Though performed often, the ovariohysterectomy surgery in humans is a major abdominal surgical procedure requiring removal of three major organs and the ligation, or tying-off, of four major blood vessel groups. In human surgery, it usually involves a large surgical team with a chief surgeon, assistant surgeon and/or resident, plus one or more skilled surgical nurses. At the Guelph Animal Hospital, Dr. Hawkins performed several of these surgeries per week with just one assistant. In most private veterinary practices, this procedure is commonly performed with just one surgeon and a circulating nurse/anesthetist. This came as a shock to me; in our surgical classes, we had a large team. But this was impractical in the real world of private practice. Likewise, Dr. Hawkins often completed these procedures in less than fifteen minutes from start to finish, whereas in our surgery classes, such surgery required at least an hour. Even allowing for our inexperience, Dr. Hawkins' surgical skill seemed extraordinary; I hoped one day to emulate his expertise.

I am often asked how a single veterinary surgeon can perform a surgery that in the human field involves much greater care. In veterinary medicine we use the neat little word "spay," and we tend to think of it as routine. It must be the sheer familiarity and the frequency with which we perform it, that allows us a relatively casual attitude. As well, our patients are usually young, healthy, and without self-pity. They don't realize they have had major surgery and must heal and recuperate.

My experience with Dr. Hawkins was an ideal complement to the next two years of predominantly clinical studies, in both companion and farm animal medicine and surgery. Our classwork supported the clinical cases. At last, all the hours of study began to make sense. My classmates and I found ourselves quoting from texts and lecture notes. We could think through our cases along with our professors. Though we were not yet professional colleagues, we were learning to think like veterinarians.

Each professor had his or her individual style and method, which often reflected the college from which they had graduated. Regardless of their ap-proach, they were all deserving of great respect because they had become ex-perts in their field. They knew more about their specific area of the profession than other veterinarians and were at the Ontario Veterinary College to communicate this expertise to us. I am not ashamed to say, more than thirty-five years after graduating, that I idealized these professors and held them up to such high standards, I was ready to accept almost any pronouncement they might make.

It was therefore shocking when Dr. Frank Milne, professor of equine surgery, who was wishing to emphasize the exacting nature and difficulty of surgery on horses, prefaced his first lecture with, "Now boys [there were three women in our class], I want you to remember that in equine surgery 99-percent success equals failure." Did Dr. Milne mean that unless we could be sure of a perfectly successful outcome we should not attempt or recommend surgery in horses? If that was true, what was our education all about? Dr. Milne was not the only professor who surprised us.

Dr. Klaus Funk, professor of large animal medicine, had many of us in awe of his case write-ups. To read his progress notes was like reading a textbook. I clearly remember one of his cases involving a rather obstreperous horse with a serious wound on the lower end of a foreleg. Treatment involved changing the wound dressing daily. As is frequently the case in veterinary medicine, the patient was his own worst enemy and became more and more difficult to treat. Finally one day Dr. Funk's progress note read, "Neither with love nor compulsion were we able to change the dressing." Was there any more eloquent and completely descriptive way to communicate the fact that this patient needed sedation to accomplish the required treatment?

For some reason, probably out of sheer contrast with the westerners in our class, Dr. Don Horney—along with some of the other large (farm) animal faculty—had decided that Steven Metz was a city boy and was neither accustomed to nor competent with horses and cattle. I displeased Dr. Horney when he asked me to give an intravenous injection of a tranquilizer to a horse in preparation for some surgery. I selected a small-sized needle (22-gauge) and gently inserted it into the large jugular vein in the horse's neck. The usual technique for the procedure was to use a much larger needle (18-gauge) and insert it with a firm "clap." My excessively delicate technique confirmed Dr. Horney's opinion that I was not cut out for working with large animals; in an attempt to instill the proper decisiveness in my technique, and being a plainspoken man, he bellowed from across the room, "Damn it, Metz—hit it!" I grabbed an 18-gauge needle and promptly plunged it into the carotid artery, too deep in the horse's neck tissue. Instead of a steady flow of blood from the needle, I got a pulsing spurt, clearly indicating my needle was in an artery instead of a vein.

Despite my profound respect for the faculty of the Ontario Veterinary College, I resented Dr. Horney's assumption that I was incompetent just because my method was different from what he was accustomed to seeing. In that instant I decided to throw a scare into him, so I began to attach the syringe full of tranquilizer to the needle as if I were about to give the drug into the artery. The carotid artery goes directly to the brain, and if I had given the injection I might well have killed the horse. When Dr. Horney saw what he thought was an impending disaster, he sprinted across the room and snatched the syringe from my hand, "What the hell are you doing?" he yelled. I might have apologized, but instead reminded him, "You said to hit it so that's what I did." I cannot recall the outcome of this exchange; however, I do recall I was not expelled from class, and Dr. Horney and I remained on speaking terms.

In addition to instruction on the premises, Ontario Veterinary College operated an ambulatory service by which students, usually two or three at a time, accompanied a professor on farm calls. This way, students had the opportunity to see firsthand the great variety of conditions under which some of our farm patients lived. These conditions played a critical part in our diagnosis and treatment of the animals. Several professors took turns with this service so we were exposed to differing approaches and techniques. The job of the student was to conduct an examination of the cow, horse, or pig (the usual farm species we saw), arrive at, or make a plan for achieving a diagnosis, and present this to the professor. Sometimes this was all done in front of the farmer and lively discussions frequently took place in the car after we left the farm. I particularly recall riding with Dr. Jack Cote several times on this ambulatory service. He was an energetic and sometimes brusque teacher. I overwhelmed him with question after question, almost as I had my grandfather so many years ago. I forced him to substantiate every diagnosis, every treatment decision. One day the harried Dr. Cote turned to me and said, "Boy, you can really talk!" Imagine my surprise when after all that pestering, Dr. Cote presented me with the Frank J. Cote Memorial Award for excellence in small animal medicine at graduation.

One final examination in clinical medicine was given by Dr. Jim Lennox; unlike many of our professors, he had been a private practitioner for several years before teaching. Dr. Lennox's teaching perspective was that of practicality—real world veterinary medicine versus the purely academic approach taught by some professors who had spent their entire careers in the hallowed halls of university. In this particular exam, Dr. Lennox required us to perform a complete physical examination of a canine patient. (The patient happened to be a friendly adult male boxer; I felt right at home.) We were to discover what—if anything— was wrong with this dog, and report the findings along with a treatment plan to Dr. Lennox. Here we were, bright young students newly equipped with our own stethoscopes, ophthalmoscopes, otoscopes, and reflex hammers, filled with knowledge, and eager to prove that we were now ready to launch ourselves into our chosen profession. Each of us was sure we would discover from what mysterious condition or disease the patient was suffering. Every one of us approached the friendly, alert dog and peered into his eyes with our ophthalmoscopes, looked deeply into his ear canals with our otoscopes, tested his reflexes with our rubber hammers, listened intently to his heartbeat and the soft, almost inaudible breathing sounds of lungs filling and emptying. We went over every inch of the dog. Student after student came away shaking their head: nothing. We could find nothing wrong with the dog. It must be a trick! Dr. Lennox was trying to trick us, trying to catch us manufacturing a problem where none existed, attempting to see if we could recognize a healthy dog after all the hours of studying disease. Still, we just weren't sure.

I can't speak for my classmates because each examination and report was done separately; none of us knew the outcome of another student's test. When it came my turn, I performed the same physical examination as all the others and, like them, found nothing obviously wrong with the dog. But somehow, I just couldn't believe the finding of a completely healthy patient. I had noticed a patch of skin over one eye where the hair seemed to be slightly thinner than all the other areas of the head. Surely, such an insignificant finding couldn't be worth mentioning on a final exam. The answer had to be something worthy of the occasion, I believed.

I went to Dr. Lennox's desk feeling a sense of failure as I reported to him that I had found an essentially healthy dog. I remember watching an expression of exasperation come over his face as he listened to my report. At the very end, as an aside and with full expectation that I would be told to concentrate on the important and obvious problems I had missed, I mentioned the small patch of thinning hair over the dog's eye. Instantly, Dr. Lennox reached out, grabbed my shoulders and gave me a shake, saying "Don't you forget it, mister. Don't ever neglect standing back and looking at the whole patient. That dog is in the early stages of demodectic mange." With great wisdom, Dr. Lennox had selected the most basic element of clinical medicine—the physical examination—and driven home its importance.

Dr. Lennox didn't know it at the time, but his admonition to our class to look at the whole patient was a precursor to an approach to medicine, both veterinary and human, that is widely popular today: holistic medicine. In my opinion, no skilled physician or veterinarian practices anything else.

Meanwhile, I was learning other valuable lessons outside our OVC classrooms. In our hamlet of Eden Mills, word had spread that I was studying veterinary medicine. One evening after class Connie and I had visitors. A young couple who had recently moved to Eden Mills introduced themselves and revealed that the wife was expecting a baby in a few months. They explained at some length that they didn't believe in hospitals and wanted their baby to be born by natural methods right in their home in Eden Mills. They didn't believe there would be any difficulties or complications and they realized I was not a physician. They had come to ask me if I would be willing to help with the birth in case any problems arose. When I recovered from this startlingly naive request, I assured the couple I would be most happy to help. I would immediately call for a taxi or ambulance, whichever seemed most appropriate at the time. This kind of help was not what they were looking for, and I did my very best to explain that if there were any complications they would absolutely require a hospital and a doctor. I made no progress, I'm afraid, and the couple left greatly disappointed.

Shortly after this obstetrical consultation, Connie and I were awakened in the early morning hours by Kin's barking. As I mentioned earlier, he almost never barked, so we felt something must be wrong. When I opened our front door, I immediately smelled smoke. Sure enough, the old mill just down the lane was on fire. Flames were shooting into the air, and one or two nearby neighbors were watching the fire from a safe distance. Eden Mills did not have its own fire department. The nearest were the city of Guelph some eight miles away, and the small town of Rockwood, an equal distance in the opposite direction. Both fire departments eventually arrived at the scene. Until then, the nearest neighbors to the mill rigged garden hoses to wet down the closest homes as well as a propane gas tank right next to the mill that we feared would explode when it got hot enough. All the residents took turns with the available hoses and pitched in when the fire departments arrived.

Our house was fairly close to the mill, so it is not impossible that sparks could have ignited our roof. The propane tank, if it exploded, could have caused damage to the house and to us. This was the second time Kin had alerted us to danger. There were two more times—one when a prisoner had escaped from the Guelph jail. He ran past our house early one morning to hide in the woods behind our field. He was recaptured thanks to Kin's alert: We saw the escapee as he ran by and pointed the police in his direction.

Kin's fourth warning highlights human carelessness that almost cost the life of a pet not supervised properly. One late winter evening as we were going to bed, Kin started to bark. By now, we had learned to pay attention. Connie opened the front door but could see no one. However, a strange half-gasping, half-crying sound was heard from the river pond just down the hill from our house. At first, we thought it might be some wild animal doing some night foraging, but the sound continued. Connie and I went cautiously down the hill to the edge of the frozen pond. The pond was actually part of a river so the ice was sometimes thin, especially in the late winter when the temperatures started to warm. There, halfway across the pond, was Pandora, our neighbor's Saint Bernard, desperately trying to claw her way back up onto the ice from a hole she had fallen into. She kept slipping all the way back into the water, submerging her head. There was no time to get any apparatus or any other help. I cautiously tested the ice, lay down on my belly, and crawled out to the edge of the hole. I didn't exactly plan how I was going to help Pandora, but thought maybe an extra tug might give her the traction she needed to get up out of the water. Her weight combined with mine could very well break the ice again—and we would both be in the water.

I reached out with one arm, grabbed a handful of the scruff of Pandora's neck, and heaved. Somehow, she got up onto the ice and collapsed completely with her back legs still dangling over the edge of the hole. She was soaking wet and utterly exhausted, unable to walk. The ice around me was cracking and sagging. Not daring to stand, I held on to the scruff of her neck and inched backwards until we got closer to shore where Connie was able to help. We had to carry Pandora to her house—a considerable task with a Saint Bernard who weighed 135 pounds dry. Her owners were away until late that night. We grabbed all the towels we could find and started vigorously drying Pandora. She was so cold at first; she couldn't even shiver.

After three quarters of an hour of drying her off and giving her continual rubdowns, Pandora was able to stand, wag her tail, and give us both a series of slobbery kisses. When her owners returned home, they were surprised to find Pandora confined to the house and a large pile of wet towels in their laundry room. They also found the note we left detailing what their dog had been through. They were very grateful, but the next day Pandora was playing outside unsupervised as before. The husband explained to me that she had undoubtedly learned her lesson and would never again go out onto the ice. I placed the same credence in that statement as I do today when I listen to an owner whose dog has just been sprayed by a skunk or quilled by a porcupine. They contend they don't have to supervise their dogs because they've learned their lesson. These dogs invariably come back time after time, having attempted to even the score.

Whether it was Pandora's intelligence or some other reason, she never again ventured out onto the ice the rest of that winter or the next. We did not maintain contact with Pandora and her family when we moved away from Eden Mills, but looking back over that episode, I still wonder how I was able to lift, even partially, a soaking wet 135-pound dog with one arm. There must be something to the theory that with enough adrenaline, you can perform tasks that would ordinarily be impossible.

Life as a veterinary student was anything but dull, both in class and out. To add excitement, two significant events occurred during my third year. In April, just before final exams, our first child Andrew was born. This occurrence was totally incompatible with serious study, and I was thankful that most of our curriculum was now actual clinical study rather than classroom work. However, there was at least one written exam on which I remember having done quite miserably. Perhaps my last page was what got me the passing grade: a cigar taped to the page with "It's a boy!" written in large letters.

Andrew survived our typical first-time parenting ineptness and because of excellent help in our Eden Mills/Guelph community, I was able to accept an offer at the end of the summer of my third year from Dr. Cliff Lobaugh up in Juneau, Alaska. He wanted to take a vacation to retrace the famous and de-manding Klondike gold rush hiking route over the Chilkoot Pass, but couldn't find a fill-in veterinarian. Unbeknownst to me, Dr. Lobaugh thought that I had just graduated from school that spring; thus, I would be qualified to manage the practice while he was away for three weeks. Given my infatuation with Alaska, I couldn't say yes fast enough. I cautioned him that most of my experience (in-cluding the two summers working for Dr. Norm Hawkins) was with compan-ion animals, rather than farm animals or horses. He assured me that no more dairy cows resided in Juneau, and although he did have a small equine practice he would take care of all the routine horse work before I came. I promised to bring him a portable anesthesia machine and demonstrate the newest meth-ods of inhalation anesthesia. He was still using injectable sodium pentothal, and I was excited about the opportunity to revolutionize his surgery practice. I prevailed on the manufacturer of the portable halothane anesthesia machine to let me take a loaner to Alaska and then had to overcome the considerable suspicion of both the Canadian and U.S. Customs officials. I did indeed arrive in Juneau on time and with the new anesthesia machine.

I anticipated a few leisurely days spent with Dr. Lobaugh at his Southeast Alaska Veterinary Clinic demonstrating the inhalation anesthesia technique to him and familiarizing myself with his drugs and equipment—some of which was considerably different from what I was used to. But within two hours of my arrival, Dr. Lobaugh was off for his wilderness odyssey. He was considerably shaken to discover that I was not a graduate veterinarian and therefore not legally qualified to perform diagnostics, prescribe or dispense medication, or perform surgery. I was equally taken aback to find that for the next two weeks I was the veterinarian for all of Juneau, Alaska, and for many miles around.

I should explain that since he had been the only veterinarian in all of southeastern Alaska, Dr. Lobaugh had a system whereby pet owners shipped their dogs and cats to him (in suitable pet carriers, of course) via the small passenger planes that connected the logging camps, fishing villages, and the few small towns in that part of the state. He would perform whatever surgery or diagnostics required and return the pet to the owner the same way. Sometimes these procedures were scheduled in advance and sometimes a surprise arrived at the Juneau airport; Dr. Lobaugh would get a call to come pick up a sick pet.

Dr. Lobaugh assured me things would go fine, but it was entirely possible that I would be presented with some challenges over the coming weeks. Thanks to my experience with Dr. Hawkins, I had actually done some surgery—under his direct supervision, of course. I would not hesitate to call one of my professors for help with a diagnosis. I was cautiously optimistic that I would not commit any drastic blunders. How Dr. Lobaugh felt about the situation I wasn't sure, but he was completely encouraging, and departed a few hours later right on schedule.

The rest of that first day passed uneventfully with just a few routine dog and cat examination and vaccination visits. Some owners were surprised to see a new face but everyone seemed to accept my substitution with good grace. I began to relax and enjoy the experience of managing a veterinary practice— something I hoped to do on my own in just a few years.

As I was opening the clinic the next morning, a worried-looking man walked in and asked for Dr. Lobaugh. I told him that Dr. Lobaugh was on vacation, and that I was filling in. "Can I help?" I asked. He said he sure hoped so because he thought that Henry, his thirty-year-old mule, had tetanus. He added that Henry was the mascot of the city of Juneau, and nothing must happen to him. My heart jumped to my throat. The very thing I feared most had happened! Certainly we were taught equine medicine in our classes and practical exercises, but my actual experience in that field didn't compare with my experience and knowledge in dog and cat medicine.

To make matters worse, the diagnosis of tetanus is not always straightforward. Members of the horse family are acutely sensitive to the tetanus toxin. This fact is one of the great ironies of nature: Horses carry the tetanus bacteria (Clostridium tetani) in their own intestine, where it does no harm—unless a wound on the horse is contaminated with soil where horse manure has been passed. The same is true of humans: The tetanus bacterium is in the soil where it survives for long periods, and any contaminated wound could lead to a case of tetanus. That is why we are vaccinated periodically throughout our lives against tetanus. Horses are vaccinated every year because of their great susceptibility to the disease.

For those who may be unfamiliar with tetanus—fortunately it is relatively rare in countries where vaccine is given—the poison made by the Clostridium bacterium changes conditions at the nerve-muscle connections throughout the body so muscles cannot relax. Instead, they go into rigid spasms, hence the term "lockjaw." Eventually, in a severe case, the breathing muscles go into spasm and the patient suffocates while fully conscious; it is a horrible disease. Members of the horse family are so sensitive to the toxin, that most cases in horses are severe. Once the toxin is in the patient's system, there is no direct treatment. All that can be done is to give tetanus antitoxin, which neutralizes further production of the toxin; give antibiotics (usually penicillin) to kill any bacteria left alive in the patient's body, presumably at the site of the wound; administer muscle relaxants and tranquilizers to minimize muscle spasms; and keep the patient nourished and hydrated while the toxin wears off. This latter objective is often quite difficult, because the jaw muscles are some of the first to go into spasm, so the patient cannot open his or her mouth to eat or drink.

The first question I asked the owner of Henry the mule was, "When was his last tetanus vaccine?" It was such widespread practice to vaccinate against tetanus yearly that I expected the answer to be something like "within the past year or two." Much to my surprise, the owner said Henry never had received a tetanus vaccination—nor did Dr. Lobaugh recommend it, because tetanus had never been found or diagnosed in the state of Alaska.

I thought to myself, You're a newcomer here, you're not an authority on equine diseases. There must be a good reason why tetanus vaccines are not being given. I was also skeptical of the owner's diagnosis. This was 1969, well before the Internet, where pet owners can now look up and get information on almost any disease. Without voicing my skepticism, I accompanied Henry's owner to a small barn just on the edge of town, where the news of Henry's illness had already spread to several young Juneau horse owners, some of whose horses were stabled in that same barn.

Hoping the owner was wrong, I examined Henry and found he could not open his mouth very much and was grinding his teeth in an attempt to chew. His gait was stiff-legged, and when I clapped my hands sharply, his whole body seemed to stiffen. Remembering that tetanus had to be the result of a contaminated wound (the owner could not remember any) I went over his entire body. Sure enough, I found a mostly healed scrape on the top of his neck just behind the back of his skull. Thinking back, the owner now remembered this insignificant-looking wound from three weeks ago. He thought it was from Henry's leather halter rubbing against the skin. He had not treated the wound in any way and it seemed to be healing normally.

Now we had a suspicious wound, an unvaccinated mule, and clinical signs compatible with tetanus. It seemed sensible to try treatment first—then argue later about whether tetanus bacterium was or was not in Alaskan soil. I administered a large dose of penicillin (still the best choice in cases of tetanus) and acepromazine, a tranquilizer. I also wanted to feed Henry, which I was going to have to do via stomach tube, and I wanted to give the prescribed dosage of tetanus antitoxin. I went back to the clinic and found a suitable horse stomach tube, routinely used for giving deworming medications to horses, but search as I might, I could not find any antitoxin. I would have to order it, and in a big hurry, if it was going to do any good.

I went through Dr. Lobaugh's files and found the name of a medical supplier he used down in Seattle. When I got them on the phone and said what I needed, they informed me that all they had were small vials, and I would need about thirty to make the dose I needed. The cost was going to be several hundred dollars plus the charge for next day air shipment. I consulted Henry's owner, and although he was not a wealthy man, he gave permission to place the order.

Meanwhile, the tube feeding needed to be done. Thank goodness I had practiced this several times at school and seemed to have the knack. Two difficulties can arise with the procedure: You must be sure to get the tube down the esophagus, not the windpipe, or the horse could drown. And if the horse is not reasonably cooperative and fights the tube, a severe nosebleed can result. A sizeable audience had now collected at Henry's barn. I was nervous enough even without the onlookers, but the procedure went smoothly, and Henry was surprisingly cooperative—possibly influenced by the tranquilizer I had given him earlier. He seemed to be resting comfortably, so I left Henry, promising to come back later that afternoon. I cautioned the owner to keep visitors away and keep things quiet around the barn; this would help minimize muscle spasms.

The rest of the morning was quiet at the clinic—leaving me lots of time to question my diagnosis. What if Henry did not have tetanus, but had some other neurological disorder that I just didn't have enough experience to diagnose? What if it were true that the tetanus bacterium did not exist in Alaska's soil? It was, I felt, a terrible coincidence that Dr. Lobaugh had spent so many years treating his horse patients without a similar problem, and my first day in Juneau turned up a case of a previously undiagnosed disease!

There were other implications to the tetanus diagnosis that I hadn't considered until my telephone began to ring: "Dr. Metz?" I hadn't the nerve to correct the caller about my lack of a degree, so I answered affirmatively. The call was from the mother of the teenage girl whose horse was stabled right next to Henry; she had been one of the observers that morning. She was concerned about her daughter. Could her daughter catch tetanus from handling Henry? I explained that one gets tetanus from a wound that has been contaminated and not cleaned or treated properly. I also suggested that her daughter had probably been vaccinated against tetanus, but that she should check with her pediatrician or family doctor. As far as I knew, children were (and still are) given a series of "DPT" vaccinations when they are young: "D" for diphtheria, "P" for pertussis, and "T" for tetanus. After this morning's revelation that horses in Alaska were not vaccinated against tetanus, I instantly regretted voicing that suggestion. After all, it was bad enough that I was questioning standard veterinary practice. I certainly didn't need to antagonize Juneau's physicians. All the while, I kept thinking, Metz, you don't even have your degree yet! What have you gotten yourself into?

Having at least been partly reassured about her daughter, the mother now began to question me about why her daughter's horse, and those of all her daughter's friends, had not been vaccinated against tetanus. I repeated what Henry's owner had told me: supposedly, there was no tetanus in Alaska. Finally came the questions I most dreaded: "Are you sure Henry has tetanus?" and worst of all, "How many of these cases have you seen, Dr. Metz?" By this time I would gladly have blurted out that I was not Dr. Metz; I was only fourth-year veterinary student Metz. However, I thought this would have gotten Dr. Lobaugh into a lot of trouble. So I answered as truthfully and accurately as I could by saying, "No, I am not sure that Henry has tetanus, but the signs are very suspicious." I mentioned that because tetanus was quite rare due to the common vaccination procedures in Ontario (and everywhere else I had been), I had actually never seen a clinical case. This was definitely not reassuring to the parent, but it was the truth, as far as I could tell it.

For the rest of the afternoon, I received calls from parents of children with horses in the Juneau area—more than a dozen calls. Evidently, word was spreading rapidly about the new disease and the new "doctor." Some parents were openly skeptical about both my diagnosis and my credentials; some wanted immediate tetanus vaccination for their horses, which was not available in Dr. Lobaugh's pharmacy. If I could be more certain of the diagnosis, I could speak with more confidence. I scoured Dr. Lobaugh's equine medicine references, looking for another possible diagnosis. From everything I read, the most likely problem was indeed tetanus. It was too late to call the Ontario Veterinary College by that time, but I determined to make the call next day.

In the morning I treated Henry again, but his signs were worse. His jaw was clenched more tightly, and he was barely able to walk. I went back to the clinic and was preparing to call my veterinary college when the door opened and a very smartly dressed gentleman walked in and asked for Dr. Lobaugh. I explained that he was on vacation and asked if I could help. He introduced himself as Dr. Fred Sattler, a veterinarian from California, who was flying his own airplane up to Anchorage for a veterinary meeting.

I almost hugged the man. Dr. Fred Sattler was one of the most famous veterinarians in the United States. His knowledge of intensive care and emergency medicine was respected and admired throughout the country and he had personally helped set up the emergency and intensive care departments for one California medical school—in human medicine. I had certainly heard of him and read some of his published articles.

The doctor listened to my tale of woe, and then, bless him, he volunteered to come see Henry. In a dress-suit, shirt, tie, and polished shoes, he performed a physical exam on Henry under the watchful eye of the gallery of young horse owners and their parents. Emerging from the stall, Dr. Sattler announced for all to hear, "Looks like tetanus to me," which obviously bolstered my standing among the onlookers.

We discussed treatment, and Dr. Sattler mentioned one additional therapy. We had both noticed that Henry was starting to accumulate some fluid in his throat, probably because his swallowing muscles weren't working properly. This fluid could pool in his lungs and lead to pneumonia, so Dr. Sattler went over the procedure for suctioning the fluid off. I would just need to get a portable suction apparatus, which should be available, said Dr. Sattler, from the local fire department. As he left to continue his trip to Anchorage, he brushed off my thanks and said, "Stick to your guns, young fellow. Just because you don't yet have your degree doesn't mean your diagnosis and treatment are wrong. That mule is lucky you're around."

I felt like a million dollars! The support of someone of Dr. Fred Sattler's stature meant everything to me. I planned to continue doing everything I could for Henry. I contacted the Juneau Fire Department and explained my need for their portable suction apparatus. The dispatcher promised to discuss my request with the chief and get back to me.

When the telephone rang I identified myself as Steven Metz (I didn't say "Doctor") and asked how I could be of help. The caller identified himself as a member of the Alaska Department of Public Health. He asked if I was the veterinarian who had just diagnosed a case of tetanus in Juneau. I said, "Yes." He then asked, "Are you aware that a soil survey of the entire state was done and no tetanus organisms were found anywhere?" I admitted to having heard that. His next remark was, "Well, then, your diagnosis must be incorrect."

Admittedly, if I had not just had the visit from Dr. Sattler, I might have gone along meekly with that premise, especially given my lack of veterinary degree. However, this doctor was in Anchorage, many miles away, and I had been examining and treating a live patient for the last two days. So I replied, "The history and clinical picture all fit the diagnosis perfectly, Doctor. May I ask when your soil survey was done?" He hemmed and hawed, then admitted it had been conducted in 1934. I hardly needed to remind him that many new horses had been brought into the state since then, each one a potential carrier of the tetanus organism, especially in a relatively densely populated area such as Juneau.

He growled, "Make sure you document everything thoroughly, Doctor," and hung up. I didn't exactly know what was meant by documenting everything thoroughly, but I certainly wrote down everything I saw, every treatment and drug I administered, and especially the visit and examination by Dr. Sattler.

By this time, many Juneau non-horse owners were getting interested in

Henry's plight, and the telephone rang more than ever. I had to leave the clinic to pick up the tetanus antitoxin I had ordered the previous day. When I got it from the freight office, I headed directly over to Henry's barn and administered the required dose. This was a vital part of the treatment, and I had high hopes that Henry would respond. I noticed he was weaker on his legs and the fluid in his throat seemed to be getting worse. I needed that suction apparatus!

Unfortunately, just as I was arriving back at the clinic, the fire chief called to explain he could not risk contaminating the fire department's equipment by using it on a sick mule. I tried to explain that Henry was not contagious, but to no avail. Meanwhile, Henry had just fallen in his stall. With help, Henry's owner had successfully gotten him back on his feet, but he was afraid he would fall again any minute. I instructed him on how to rig a sling for Henry and told him I'd come right back over.

By this time it was mid-afternoon and I felt exhausted. It seemed I'd been in continual motion since first thing in the morning, and I'd definitely spent more time in Henry's barn than in the Southeast Alaska Veterinary Clinic. I recalled Dr. Lobaugh's description of what my two weeks would be like: an hour or two in the clinic in the morning, then fishing, hiking, or boating the rest of the day. It would really be a vacation for me, said Dr. Lobaugh.

In stark contrast to that pronouncement, the next several days were a blur. I don't remember much about the other pets I saw, but I clearly remember poor Henry getting weaker and weaker despite everything I tried. I was at the barn every spare moment; Henry's owner spent as much time consoling me as feeling bad about his mule. We both gradually came to grips with the possibility of having to euthanize Henry—or to use the more popular euphemism, "put him down." Before we had to take that step, Henry took the decision out of our hands and passed quietly away during the night.

I never thought about a necropsy (the veterinary equivalent of an autopsy) to confirm the diagnosis of tetanus. This would have been very difficult, even for a skilled pathologist; unlike many other diseases, the tetanus toxin does not cause noticeable organ damage. Thus Henry the mule, mascot of Juneau, was buried with a small ceremony attended by his friends and one veterinary student who kept asking himself, What more could I have done?

The rest of my stay at the Southeast Alaska Veterinary Clinic was uneventful, and Dr. Lobaugh returned just one day before I was due to leave. I tried to explain that in his absence I had diagnosed and attempted unsuccessfully to treat a disease that was not believed to exist in his entire state. I also tried to warn him that authorities from the Alaska Department of Public Health had questioned my diagnosis (and my identity); additionally, many of his clients were now wondering why he had not vaccinated their horses and ponies, and were clamoring for vaccinations before their animals contracted this obviously deadly disease.

In his easy-going way (after all, he had just come back from a wonderful vacation) Dr. Lobaugh tried to calm me down. It would all blow over, he said. I strongly believe to this day he doubts the diagnosis. In 1982 I took our family on a camping trip and visited him. When I spoke to him on the telephone in the summer of 2006, he remembered the incident clearly. His memory is not what it used to be, so I can only surmise that there must have been a significant uproar straightening out the fuss I left behind.

As for my reminder of Henry the mule, I have only to look at the bookshelf behind my desk to see an exquisite and valuable ivory carving of an Eskimo hunter confronting a polar bear. Henry's owner along with some of Henry's friends presented this most treasured memento to me at the clinic as I was packing to leave. I remember feeling stunned that I was being given a treasured gift for caring for a patient I had not saved. In my mind, I didn't deserve a gift; I might have expected an admonishment (if not outright blame) for not having been able to see Henry through his illness.

When I returned to Connie and Andrew in Eden Mills, I confess I felt as if a weight had been lifted from me. The responsibility of Dr. Lobaugh's practice, particularly because I had not yet actually earned the right to undertake that responsibility, had been heavy. If ever I hoped to open my own practice, I would certainly have to learn to cope with the pressures and stress that go hand-in-hand with the profession.

chapter four

From Learning to Practice

A s I began my senior year at Ontario Veterinary College, the question of what to do next was easily answered by some in my class. They would go home and join a practice where they had already been working. With few exceptions, all of us were planning to become private practitioners rather than work for the government or in a research laboratory, although our education qualified us to do so. Where would Connie, Andrew, Kin, and I go? Would we stay in Canada? Would we consider life in the West, especially in the Northwest—Alaska for example? A large part of that decision would depend upon my ability to pass the state or provincial examinations given to every graduate to ensure competency. In my day in veterinary medicine, a new graduate had to take an extensive written examination recognized by all the states, and then a practical examination in the state where that graduate was applying for a license. These examinations tested material from our entire education, from basic physiology, microscopic histology, and animal science, to the latest medical and surgical procedures. They are equivalent to a lawyer passing the bar exam or a human physician becoming licensed to practice medicine. Some of these examinations took as long as forty-eight hours.

We all hoped our education had equipped us for these examinations because failure meant we could not accept a position or practice until we could attempt them again several months later. We therefore proceeded on the assumption that we would pass the exams, and began our search for positions. My strong feeling was that, as rigorous and complete as our Ontario Veterinary College experience had been, we still had a tremendous amount to learn. I felt that an internship would prepare me for the real world of veterinary practice. After briefly considering equine practice I decided that the challenge of companion animal medicine was where my fascination lay. It was called small animal medicine at that time, although there is nothing small about a 211-pound English mastiff. Companion animal medicine held fewer financial constraints on the care of a pet versus a farm animal, where the veterinarian is obligated to consider the commercial value of the patient before recommending treatment.

To see a large number of cases with the most advanced medicine and surgery being practiced, I would have to seek a position in or near a large city. Both Connie's and my family were in Massachusetts, so we decided that New England, or at least the Northeast, was our first choice. For the immediate future, I gave up my dream of returning to Alaska or the Northwest provinces. Upon one thing I was firmly resolved: Family or no family, I would never practice in Massachusetts! I would not even apply for a license. The memory of Dean Armistead's words about taking Massachusetts castoffs haunts me to this day.

Once these two fundamental decisions were made, I began to look at available positions in the metropolitan New York-New Jersey area, reasoning that along with large, affluent population centers came busy, sophisticated veterinary practices that would provide the best opportunity for associating with the most accomplished practitioners and learning all the latest techniques. I had to swallow hard when I thought of living in a city after three and a half years in Ketchikan, Alaska, population 7,000; four years in Guelph Ontario, population 49,000; and Eden Mills, just 40. Connie, bless her, seemed willing to go along with this plan. One week near the end of our final semester, I flew into New York City and began a round of twenty-one interviews at veterinary hospitals from the middle of New Jersey to the tip of Long Island, New York. I met many veterinarians, some friendly and outgoing, some rather formal and stand-offish. At some interviews I was treated as a colleague, while at others I was regarded as a student. The veterinary hospitals were as different from one another as were their owners. Some had several veterinarians on staff and some were solo practices. The facilities and equipment varied greatly from hospital to hospital. Likewise, the requirements and qualifications for positions at different hospitals varied. One practitioner was looking for another veterinarian so he could semi-retire and spend less time in the practice, while other practices needed to add a veterinarian because of rapid growth.

It was a great learning experience because my contact with veterinarians and hospitals had been limited, at one end of the spectrum, to the Ontario Veterinary College—with every instrument and drug readily available—and at the other, the one-doctor Guelph Animal Hospital.

For my interviews, I compiled a list of several key questions that would help me choose an appropriate first position:

1) Did the veterinarian(s) at the practice seem concerned with practicing state-of-the-art medicine and surgery?

2) Was continuing education of the veterinary and nursing staff emphasized and encouraged?

3) Did the atmosphere in the practice seem conducive to teaching a new graduate the art as well as the science of veterinary practice?

4) Was the physical set up of the hospital and equipment commensurate with the practice of high quality medicine and surgery?

Notice the absence of a question about salary and benefits. Call it naive, unrealistic, or idealistic, but I truly did not ask about these issues. I knew I had a lot to learn as a new graduate, and as long as the salary was sufficient to allow reasonable living for my new son, my wife, and me, I would be quite satisfied— provided the teaching/learning opportunity existed in that practice. Now that I have been on the other side of the fence for several decades, the employer side, I can tell you that this attitude is certainly not the prevailing one. I have interviewed applicants who placed salary and benefits above all other points of discussion in the interview.

While I was being interviewed, however, I was also conducting my own interview. Toward the end of this whirlwind week of visits and interviews, three practices particularly stood out in my mind. At a practice in Riverhead, Long Island, I was interviewed by Dr. Ingram, who was unusually personable and interested in my goal of furthering my education. He thought the practice in Riverhead would be ideal for that purpose. Riverhead seemed far enough away from New York City to be a pleasant living circumstance. There was at least one other veterinarian—the owner—whom I did not meet during the visit. When I left Dr. Ingram, I promised to speak with him further about joining the practice soon.

The second interesting practice was in a small community in northern Rhode Island owned and operated by Dr. Leo Minesce. This veterinarian had a theory of practice far ahead of its time. You did not need a veterinary degree to draw a blood sample, take a radiograph (x-ray), give injections, or master many of the other skills I had just spent four years learning. Dr. Minesce believed a well-trained veterinary nurse could perform these tasks just as well as a veterinarian, thus saving time for the doctor to use his education more properly in the actual diagnosing and treatment of diseases. In this way, one veterinarian, supported by a well-trained nursing staff, could help many more patients without having a large and far more costly veterinary staff.

This was in 1970, almost fifteen years before the appearance of veterinary technician schools that are so common today. Though this strategy is well accepted now, Dr. Minesce told me he was under much criticism from other veterinarians in Rhode Island for permitting non-veterinary staff to perform minor medical procedures (under veterinary supervision) that had been previously reserved for graduate veterinarians. Either I made a poor impression on Dr. Minesce or he was so convinced by his own theory that by the end of the interview he wasn't at all sure he really wanted an associate veterinarian.

A third practice that impressed me was also in Rhode Island: Warwick Animal Hospital—a modern, utilitarian-looking building on U.S. Route 1, Elmwood Avenue, in Warwick, Rhode Island. This practice was rapidly expanding from a three-doctor to a five-doctor hospital, making it the largest practice I visited. I walked into the reception area of the hospital deliberately a half-hour early. I wanted to see how I would be greeted by the reception staff. At one of my interviews when I came early, the receptionist told me that the doctor wasn't available and I should come back at the correct time. I wondered how the interviewing doctor at Warwick would react to having a prospective colleague in the waiting room of the hospital. Would I be left to sit and wait as if I were a client, or would I be welcomed as a fellow professional?

I was not expecting a royal welcome or that all other activity in the hospital should come to a screeching halt upon my arrival, but I have always believed that a professional colleague, even a young one, should be treated with respect. In my practice, if a veterinarian comes for a visit, even an unannounced one and even if he or she is a complete stranger, I make it a point to invite that colleague personally into the treatment area of the hospital. Likewise, if a veterinarian calls and asks to speak to me on the telephone, I try hard to come right to the phone, unless I am in the middle of a difficult appointment or an actual surgery.

At the Warwick Animal Hospital, barely two minutes went by when the door from the inner section of the hospital burst open and an extremely energetic veterinarian, Dr. James Robbin, came rushing out and took me by the arm. He quickly introduced himself, got my name, and then said, "Come into our lab. I've got to show you this!" Off we headed at a trot to the hospital laboratory, where Dr. Robbin pointed to a microscope where a slide of a blood sample was being examined by one of the practice nurses (as they were called at that time). He waited with expectation as I examined the slide. Finally, unable to hold back, he asked, "Do you see it?" I felt as if I were back in Dr. Lennox's final examination as I replied, "It looks pretty normal to me." Obviously disappointed, Dr. Robbin asked, "Don't you see the basophilic stippling of the red blood cells?" He meant by this that there were tiny little blue dots inside the red blood cells of the sample. Dr. Robbin was excited about this stippling because just one month prior, a report had been published in the Journal of the American Veterinary Medical Association identifying these dots as a sign of lead poisoning. Until that report, the usual way of diagnosing lead poisoning was by traditional analysis of a blood sample, which took several days to complete. Meanwhile the patient often suffered seizures, blindness, or other serious clinical signs. The veterinarian was forced to guess at the cause. Here at the Warwick Animal Hospital there would be no guessing—because the blood was being examined under a microscope by this conscientious, perceptive, up-to-date veterinarian.

As I was a new graduate, Dr. Robbin expected me to have all the very latest information; he hoped he and the other three veterinarians in the practice would learn from me. However, my classmates and I had been so involved in attending lectures and studying for examinations that most of us had found little time to read the latest journals and reports. Instead, we studied notes taken from our lectures and we read textbooks. As we soon discovered, the field of medicine (both veterinary and human) changes so rapidly that much of the information in our textbooks was two or more years out of date by the time the books were published. This is still true today and is the reason medicine is a lifelong study. Theories and methods accepted as state-of-the-art today may be modified or even totally disproven by the following week or month.

The next step in my interview was prefaced by an apology from Dr. Robbin, who explained that he and his partner, Dr. George Maurice, were just about to do a dissection of a dog cadaver to refresh their knowledge of the anatomy and arrangement of the blood vessels emerging from the heart. The next day they were planning to perform surgery on a young puppy that was born with a life-threatening defect in these blood vessels, called "patent ductus arteriosus." This condition allowed some of his circulating blood to bypass his lungs and thus not get a supply of oxygen. The circulation bypasses the lungs through a short blood vessel called the ductus arteriosus. When a puppy or kitten (or human baby) is born, this blood vessel is supposed to close down rapidly and no longer permit the newborn's blood to bypass the lungs.

When this dachshund puppy came to the Warwick Animal Hospital for his check-up and vaccinations a few days before my interview visit, the veterinarian who examined him heard a loud, continuous heart murmur and felt a throbbing in the puppy's chest called a thrill. These findings led to the diagnosis of patent ductus arteriosus. This was long before the veterinary specialist boom. Few veterinarians took special training in surgery or any other field for that matter, the most notable exception being pathology. There were no veterinary cardiac surgeons to refer this puppy to, as one would today. So this was a difficult surgery requiring great skill and exact knowledge of anatomy. I was extremely impressed. None of the twenty other practices I visited had been in the midst of such an undertaking.

I stood and watched as these two experienced practitioners (who had been classmates at the New York State College of Veterinary Medicine at Cornell) did a painstaking dissection of the area of the heart to prepare themselves for the next day's surgery. They could have reviewed the anatomy by using a textbook or relied on their considerable experience, but because they were both exceptional people as well as skilled, meticulous veterinarians, they took the time and made the effort to equip themselves thoroughly.

When the dissection and the accompanying discussion of the surgical procedure (which I found as fascinating and instructive as any lecture I had ever attended) was finished, Drs. Robbin and Maurice took me into the office of the hospital and commenced the formal interview. They asked the usual questions about my educational and personal background, which in those days was not prohibited as it is today. I asked many of the same questions I had asked at the previous practices.

It was plain that state-of-the-art medicine and surgery were being practiced, and continuing education was not only encouraged but absolutely necessary if you were to live up to the standards of that practice. I had already learned more in a two-hour interview at the Warwick Animal Hospital than in several hours of class and laboratory studies at the Ontario Veterinary College—all cutting edge aspects of practice. This veterinary hospital seemed the most dynamic, most exciting, most forward-thinking of all the twenty-one practices I had seen. The two partner-owners both seemed, in their separate ways, to be practitioners and persons worthy of great respect, with whom I could work and from whom I could learn. This was the practice for me, and I said so on the spot. No cagey bargaining or playing hard to get from me; this was way too important for games.

Dr. Maurice, who had a master's degree in business administration, and who delighted in challenging people, especially those who seemed sure of themselves, asked me, "Out of all those we've interviewed for this position so far, why should we choose you as our associate? What sets you apart from other applicants?"

My reply was, "My attitude towards my profession and my desire to learn and excel. I will work as conscientiously as humanly possible to become a proficient practitioner worthy of respect in this practice." I was not just saying what I thought they would like to hear. I felt an enormous respect for these two men. I wanted them as my teachers and guides along the path to becoming a skilled and respected member of my profession. I had met no one thus far of their caliber.

They asked me to retire to the reception area. When they called me back, they offered me the position. The offer was conditional on my acceptance of their salary package, and my wife's approval—and they would like to meet her as well. Until now, the question of salary had not been discussed. My primary concern was to spend my first year in a practice strongly conducive to learning. Drs. Maurice and Robbin evidently understood my priorities: Their salary offer was by far the lowest of any of the nineteen other job offers I received. The $12,500 was exactly half the salary offered by two New Jersey practices. I must have flinched visibly, because Dr. Robbin, in a fatherly way, explained that since my salary was less than that of a more experienced veterinarian (a significant understatement), he and Dr. Maurice would not begrudge spending the time necessary to teach me what I needed to become proficient. My hesitation was only momentary, and I assured the two partners I would return to Ontario, consult with my wife, and call back with an answer within forty-eight hours. I left Rhode Island and the job-hunting process in a daze.

Within two weeks, Connie and I had returned to Rhode Island, spent a relaxing evening with Jim and Shirley Robbin and George and Connie Maurice, and finalized plans for me to join the veterinary staff of the Warwick Animal Hospital. Looking back at my career, this critical choice of a first position proved to be one of the best decisions I have ever made. I have known many young veterinarians, including at least three of my classmates, who have not chosen their first practice wisely. Many promising young practitioners have been so discouraged and disillusioned by an unpleasant experience or an inconsiderate senior colleague or practice owner that they have retired from clinical practice, carrying with them a very poor opinion of the members of their chosen profession.

Some obstacles remained before I could begin at Warwick. First, I had to pass my final examinations at Ontario Veterinary College and receive my Doctor of Veterinary Medicine degree, the three precious letters—DVM—that ever afterward would follow my signature and be a symbol of fulfilled hope in my life. I was able to pass the finals and became a proud graduate DVM, Class of 1970. I was recognized for excellence in small animal medicine and I graduated fourth in my class. In the midst of the graduation ceremony, the image of the histology professor at Western Reserve University medical school and his predictions came back to me: I would never be accepted to a college of veterinary medicine; I could never complete the course; I would finish at the bottom of my class. He had been completely wrong, and I vowed never to forget the lesson of lack of humility. I also vowed to help and encourage students aspiring to enter my profession because I knew very well what it meant to receive that help—and not to receive it.

Looming even more ominously were the state or provincial examinations. These are required regardless of whether one has been awarded the Doctor of Veterinary Medicine degree; it was possible for a graduate veterinarian never be able to practice their profession. To make them even more formidable, the examinations included absolutely everything in the entire veterinary curriculum.

The first day was a written examination. The second day was practical, meaning the applicant had to perform actual tests and procedures on live animals or, as in the New York practical exam, identify various poisonous plants from dried leaves. These examinations varied tremendously in scope and difficulty. Some states made up their own examinations, from questions submitted by practitioners in that state. Others used the relatively new national exam—which was far from a national examination, as many states did not accept it. There was no reciprocity between states as there is today; thus a graduate wishing to keep future options open to practice in more than one state (in case of a move or an opportunity in another area of the country) would be required to take a separate examination for each state.

The examinations included material we had studied almost four years ago, so most of us had to do some serious reviewing—and do it while we were preparing for the final exams of our senior year at OVC. Most new graduates, at least at that time, chose to take the state exams as soon after graduation as possible, reasoning that the material would never be fresher in our minds.

Our family decision to stay in the Northeast meant that I took examinations in all the New England states except Massachusetts (despite my parents' entreaties) and New York. Taking these examinations was, in itself, an education. The first and most crucial was the Rhode Island exam, which I had to pass to accept the position at the Warwick Animal Hospital. The state of Rhode Island used the national written test, for which I was as prepared as you could be considering the scope of material.

The practical exam provided one of those unforgettable moments in my early career. An x-ray film of a dog's torso was displayed, and I was asked to comment on the film. What I didn't understand was that one of the dog's front legs was folded backward alongside the ribcage. This is an abnormal way to take a film of an animal's chest or leg; one of the cardinal rules of taking radiographs is that the film should concentrate on the area of concern without extraneous structures in the picture. The idea behind this trick radiograph, I suppose, was to test the applicant's ability to identify normal structures even if they were presented in an abnormal way. Whatever the reason, I was completely baffled. I thought perhaps it was a stick that had penetrated the skin of the dog's side or some other kind of foreign body. When I voiced that thought, the examiner asked, "Where did you say you were hoping to have a position?" I answered, "The Warwick Animal Hospital," whereupon the examiner growled, "Jim Robbin and George Maurice sure have their work cut out for them with you."

In another part of this same examination I was paired with a fellow applicant who, it turned out, was also joining the professional staff of the Warwick Animal Hospital. We were asked to do a complete physical examination of a lively young fox terrier and report our findings. One part of a standard physical examination of a dog or cat is to look into the ear canal and if possible see the tympanum, or ear drum. This requires that the patient stand reasonably still; otherwise there is a risk of injuring the ear.

Anyone familiar with the fox terrier breed can predict that the last thing this little sparkplug wanted to do was stand still while two strangers poked otoscopes deep into his ear. In fact he would have put Fred Astaire, Michael Jackson, or any break dancer to absolute shame. Thus neither my partner (and future colleague) nor I were able to examine the ears very well, much less the tympanum. When the examiner questioned us about the ears, specifically asking if we had seen the tympanum, my exam partner said he had examined the ear drum, while I said I had not been able to. For the second time that day I was the recipient of a dubious look from an examiner.

I was sorry not to have completed all aspects of the physical examination of this patient, but I was also well aware of a part of the oath I and all graduates of American and Canadian schools had taken upon receiving my degree: "First, do no harm." In my judgment, we would have hurt the terrier if we insisted on examining his ear drum—and, after all, he had probably not been consulted about volunteering to be a subject for the examination. If this had been a truly sick dog and if it were important to look at his tympanum, my preference would have been to give the little fellow a sedative first, so he wouldn't have been uncomfortable and would not have resisted so vigorously. I admit I was rather surprised, and not a little disgusted with the veterinarian with whom I would be working closely in the near future (provided I passed the exam). Surely an examiner would prefer absolute honesty and accuracy to a false answer given for the sake of passing an exam. I was careful not to give any hint about the truth of my fellow applicant's answer. In the end, this veterinarian did not fit into the professional atmosphere of the Warwick Animal Hospital and was asked to leave at the end of his one-year contract.

Two days after the Rhode Island exam, I was required to go to Hartford, Connecticut, to take that state's examination. The written exam was the national exam, which I had just taken two days before in Rhode Island; nevertheless, the Connecticut examiners insisted I repeat the test in their state. Several weeks after the Connecticut exam, I travelled to Augusta, Maine, and took the Maine exam. I don't remember much about the written Maine exam, but I clearly recall the practical examination. The examiner, a veteran practitioner, took me into an examination room of the veterinary hospital where this part of the exam was being conducted. He brought in a good-natured English bulldog, and asked me to perform a physical examination and comment on my observations as I progressed.

I had just begun my examination when the rather crusty elderly practitioner abruptly stopped me. "Enough of that. You obviously know how to examine a dog. Have a seat and a coffee and tell me why you think so many veterinarians are taking the Maine examination this year." Talk about a contrast among examinations!

In any event, I passed the Rhode Island, Connecticut, Maine, New Hampshire, and Vermont examinations—the latter being a handwritten essay test such as you might have as an undergraduate student. I postponed taking the New York state exam until the following year. The New York exams were the most grueling, exhaustive examinations I have ever taken. They were given at the veterinary college at Cornell University where I had been an undergraduate, and where I had been refused entry three times. I admit that nostalgia was not my prevailing emotion as I came back to the campus in Ithaca.

I had been warned that the New York examination was rigorous and wide-ranging. Unlike any other examination I had taken, the practical exam would include a section on identification of poisonous plants that livestock might encounter in a farm pasture. We would be asked to determine the age of horses, cattle, and sheep by looking at their teeth. We would be presented with tissue

60   S T E V E N   B .   M E T Z ,   D . V . M .

specimens from the post mortem room at the university—specimens from actual cases of disease. Veterinarians who had taken this exam told me that there was "the Cornell way" and there was everyone else's way, and an applicant had better know "the Cornell way" to pass this exam. I therefore took a week off before the exam, drove to Ithaca, and studied all the animals in the barn, hoping they would be used on the test. I reviewed the basic sciences, realizing that another full year had passed since I last studied these subjects. I especially studied all the material available on the infamous poisonous plants.

Security at this exam was extremely strict. If at any time during the course of the day, you needed a bathroom break you had to ask permission and have an escort. Box lunches were brought in so we didn't have to leave the examination area. No coffee or friendly discussion were permitted during this exam.

The material was the most difficult I had ever encountered. I recall that the leaves of the poisonous plants were dried up and shriveled—very different from the fresh young leaves from the illustrations in the books I had studied. Perhaps a professional botanist could have identified them, but in many cases my answers approached complete guesses. It seemed impossible that I could pass this section of the exam. It wasn't much consolation that all the others taking this test seemed to feel the same way. I would just have to do better on the other sections to make up for the dried leaves.

At least I could tell ages of horses and sheep, the two species on which we would be tested. I approached the first horse, who seemed agreeable, and separated his upper and lower lips so I could look for grooves in his front teeth, the angle at which the front teeth met, and the amount of general wear. Horses have grooves in their front teeth that extend from the gum line of the tooth toward the tip. The age of the horse can be determined in part by how long these grooves are and their position on the tooth. There is just one little catch: At a certain advanced age these grooves disappear entirely. This usually happens when the horse is twenty or thirty years old. None of us who had prepared for the exam imagined that the examiners would scour the barns and farms around Ithaca for horses and sheep with teeth in the worst condition possible.

"Well?" the examiner asked impatiently, looking behind me to prepare for the next victim. I could feel the sweat starting to appear on my face. There were absolutely no grooves of any length on this horse's teeth. How, then, was I supposed to tell this animal's age? Suddenly, my mind went back—more than twenty years back—to a wonderful horse story I had read as a boy, Black Beauty. The setting of this book was England during a time when horses were the primary means of transportation and were being bought and sold routinely. Determining a horse's age was routine in this book. I remembered the wonderful phrase used in Black Beauty to describe a horse whose teeth were in precisely the same condition as those of the animal I was now facing.

Releasing the horse's head, I turned to the examiner and replied, "This horse is aged. That's all that can be determined from the condition of his teeth." The examiner looked at me for a moment, then said, "There are other ways to estimate a horse's age, but basically you are exactly correct." I felt so relieved. Here was Dr. Jim Lennox's lesson all over again: Look at the whole picture; let so-called common sense prevail.

By some miracle and due in no small part to the excellent education I had received at the Ontario Veterinary College, I passed every examination I took. I was now legally able to practice veterinary medicine in any capacity I chose. I could start my own practice, I could diagnose disease problems in any animal species I encountered, and I could prescribe medication for those animals. I could operate on any patient, and I could, with the owner's consent, end an animal's life. I could do all these things regardless of my experience or lack of experience.

chapter five

The Real World of Veterinary Practice

As a new graduate, I had much to learn about the practice of veterinary medicine. My encounter with basophilic stippling of red blood cells during my interview at Warwick Animal Hospital was just one example. As I was legally qualified to do all the things a veterinarian did, it was my responsibility to make sure I was truly qualified. As it turned out, I could not have chosen a better learning environment. My wonderful mentors, Dr. Jim Robbin and Dr. George Maurice had seemingly endless patience with my inexpert methods. They used a grand combination of gentle prodding ("Same dog?" Dr. Robbin would ask during an overly lengthy surgery), pointed correction ("Do you know what is normal? How many have you seen?" asked Dr. Maurice) and, when called for, outright sarcasm. If I expressed dissatisfaction with the way a patient responded to treatment, I would be challenged: "What could you have done differently? Try the new method on the next patient."

If I wanted to change the way something was being done, I had better be sure to cite references to prove the worth of the proposed method, and if I did, I was encouraged to make the change and keep everyone informed on the results. Not all my suggestions were received gracefully. I recall asking Dr. Maurice to change the brand of cat vaccine he had been using for several years to a new brand. My reason was that the one we were using seemed to sting our kitty patients, and I didn't like that reaction. Unfortunately, the new vaccine I proposed to use cost more than twice as much. For several days afterward Dr. Maurice referred to me as the prima donna of the practice. However, we did eventually switch.

My relationship with the nurses (now called veterinary technicians) at Warwick Animal Hospital was far more complicated than with the doctors. Any new doctor will identify with my situation. I was the least experienced practitioner, clearly the low doctor on the totem pole. The nurses had more experience than I, but they were not doctors. No matter how experienced or knowledgeable they were, by law they could not diagnose, prescribe, or operate, and therefore were theoretically obliged to follow my directions, even if they believed them to be questionable or incorrect.

As a young, proud, and, yes, somewhat arrogant new doctor, I was particularly sensitive to any hint of disagreement or criticism from the nurses. There were twenty nurses and receptionists on the staff of the hospital, but I remember three in particular who used to raise my blood pressure and get my stomach churning every time I worked with them. It seemed to me they had an overly casual attitude about any directions I might give; they performed their tasks reluctantly and without conviction. I took this as criticism and lack of proper respect. I never considered that these nurses might be trying to compensate for an overly earnest, somewhat compulsive young doctor who might reassure worried pet owners by relaxing and by not taking himself so seriously.

I remember a dream I used to have that Donald Trump would surely have been proud of. In this dream I would arrive at the hospital first thing in the morning and greet the staff—including the three offenders—pleasantly, then with no change in my voice or expression I would continue my greeting by pointing to each of the three, saying "You, you, and you. You're fired!" No such thing could happen, as I was not responsible for personnel management, nor was I equipped to be at this stage of my career.

It is quite fitting then, given my feelings toward these particular nurses, that the one dog bite I have ever had on the job thus far occurred because I reacted to the casual, even careless way one of the three nurses was preparing to pick up an aggressive dog. I was sure she was about to be bitten. I quickly stepped into the examination room, stopped her, and gave her instructions on the safe way to pick up such an angry dog. Then I proceeded to demonstrate the technique—in slow motion. The slow speed gave the doggie all the opportunity he needed: He turned his head and bit down firmly on my forearm. I continued to lift the dog onto the examination table, but noticed something was bleeding profusely. The something turned out to be my arm, which had a puncture all the way through the muscle, grazing the radius bone. It was possible to take a long Q-tip and push it all the way through my arm. Forty-one years later, the scar is still visible. I was fortunate to escape any permanent nerve damage, although my hand and lower arm were numb for several days.

Many evenings I came home feeling as if no matter how hard I tried to remember everything I had learned, there would always be some important detail I overlooked. I hadn't paid enough attention to the way the sick cat was standing with her abdomen tucked up. I hadn't noticed the crusty discharge at the corners of the eyes and nose of that listless puppy. I had neglected to listen to the heart of the limping dog—paying too much attention to the apparent problem and neglecting to do a complete physical examination. Time after time, it was drilled into me to do a complete physical examination no matter why a pet was brought to me. Our patients cannot talk; they cannot tell us what's wrong or where they hurt. There is no rule that says a patient can have only one problem at a time. Dr. Maurice and Dr. Robbin continually emphasized that even if I developed into the most skilled surgeon and successfully performed spectacular procedures, if I did not do a thorough and complete physical examination, I would be endangering and short-changing my patients.

To make the transition from student to practitioner even more exciting, our daughter, Rebecca, was born only a month after I joined the staff of the Warwick Animal Hospital. Rebecca was not content with being born in Rhode Island; she joined us during a weekend trip to visit our parents in Springfield, Massachusetts. She weighed only four pounds and fourteen ounces at birth, and the doctors felt she needed to stay in the hospital in Springfield for several extra days. Fortunately, my wife's father was an M.D. and had privileges at the local hospitals, so my wife could stay with her parents. It turned out to be a thrilling weekend trip, and when we brought Rebecca home, our family life was even more busy and unpredictable.

It was a good addition to my education to realize how much veterinary patient care is not unlike the practice of pediatrics. The pediatrician must communicate with the parents of a patient; the veterinarian must do likewise with the owners of a patient. If that communication is unsuccessful, the pediatrician or the veterinarian may not get to treat the sick patient. This is the art of medical practice, both veterinary and human. Yet we receive almost no training at medical school in that art. Within one month of joining the Warwick Animal Hospital, I had an experience that underlined the importance of this art of communication.

After-hours emergencies were seen and cared for by whichever veterinarian was on call. That veterinarian was expected to examine and provide care for any patient needing care from approximately 6 p.m. when the hospital closed until the hospital reopened at 8 a.m. There were no emergency hospitals as there are today. Dr. Maurice or Dr. Robbin were usually available by telephone, so Dr. Parker (my partner in taking the Rhode Island state examination) and Dr. Christine Seidler, the other two practitioners, often consulted with the senior partners when faced with a difficult emergency. Both Dr. Parker and Dr. Seidler had been graduate veterinarians for several years but were very glad to have help upon occasion.

I had been at Warwick for about one month when it was decided that I was ready to take call. I don't know who was more nervous as the evening approached, Drs. Maurice and Robbin or me. I left the hospital a little early so I could get dinner before what might be a long night. I remember sitting down at the table and lifting my fork for my first bite when the phone rang. A woman's voice asked, "Is this Dr. Metz?" (I was still thrilled to be addressed as Dr. Metz even four months post graduation.) I agreed to the identification, and the woman continued, "I would like you to put my dog to sleep right away. He's just bitten his third person; he's out of control, and I'm completely afraid of him." She seemed so agitated and insistent that without questioning her further, I said I would meet her at the hospital right away. So much for dinner!

In many states, you are not allowed to euthanize a domestic animal right after it has bitten someone. Instead, a quarantine period is required to see if the animal shows any signs of rabies, in which case the bitten person may well have to undergo a series of injections to prevent rabies from developing. Thus, I was determined to try to dissuade the owner from making a hasty decision. We both arrived in the hospital parking lot at the same time. As I got out of my car, I heard a loud snarl, followed by an insistent, deep-pitched barking, indicating a larger breed was the source of the sound. I turned around, and there, lunging at me from across the parking lot—which suddenly seemed quite small—was a huge, aggressive German shepherd at the end of a large chain. At the other end was a young man who looked to be about sixteen.

It was difficult to tell who was more angry, the dog or the young man. It was not difficult to see that the woman who got out of the driver's seat was frightened, upset, and determined. Because of the continuous barking and snarling, conversation in the parking lot was impossible. Once we were inside the hospital, I motioned to the young man to tie the dog to a strong doorknob with the chain. As we stepped into another examination room and closed the door, the young man exploded. Pointing his finger directly at me and only inches from my face, he said, "If you put my dog to sleep, I want you to know that I will leave home and never have anything to do with my mother again. Getting this dog was the last thing my Dad and I did together before he died, and she has always hated him. Now she is finally trying to get rid of him."

As I opened my mouth to reply, the mother turned to me and started to cry. She sobbed, "You can see what kind of dog he is, can't you, Doctor? My son

S t e v e n   B .   M e t z ,   d . v . m .

won't train him, won't keep him tied up, and this is the third person he's bitten. I can't afford to get sued, and I'm terrified of the animal."

I turned back to the son, but before I could say anything he shouted, "She's always hated this dog, even when he was a puppy! She never gave him a chance!" All this time, on the other side of the exam room wall, the barking and growling continued nonstop. I felt like a ping-pong ball. This was obviously a family conflict that had been going on for some time. These people didn't need an emergency veterinarian. They needed an emergency psychiatrist—and a wild animal trainer judging by the brief look I'd had at the object of this conflict. Nothing in my training had even remotely equipped me to deal with a situation like this. I had expected no such challenge on my first night on emergency call—or ever in my career. This was a deep-seated family conflict with serious consequences, and I had no idea how to resolve it. I couldn't even get a chance to speak. And I was beginning to get angry that these people were putting me in the middle of their family fight.

I decided to use shock tactics to stop the fighting between mother and son. Turning to the son, I raised my voice just enough to startle him, and demanded, "Do you want to save your dog's life?"

He looked at me in surprise and answered, "Sure I do."

"Then put your dog back in the car so we can have a normal conversation," I commanded.

I don't know whether it was relief that I was not going to put his dog to sleep on the spot, or whether he hadn't been spoken to in that manner in a while, but he quickly did exactly as I asked. The mother started to protest, "But, Doctor, this dog has to be put to sleep—"

I cut her off, "Do you want to lose your son?" He was still out of the room.

"No," she quavered.

"Then give me a chance to help," I said, and we waited until her son returned to the exam room.

When he did, I didn't give anyone a chance to speak. I said, "If you want me to help you, you'll have to stop shouting at each other and listen to what I have to say. If you can't do that, then please go home." Then I stopped, looked at them, and waited. After a minute the son said, "Okay, but I'm not letting her put my dog to sleep."

I ignored that and instead I asked him, "Did your dog bite someone?"

"Yes, but—"

I cut him off (I was getting better at doing that every minute). "Has he bitten people before?" The young man admitted the dog had bitten others. I asked, "Do you think that's okay for a dog to bite people—no matter what the reason?" I didn't give him a chance to answer. I continued, "I've handled hundreds of German shepherds (a significant exaggeration at this early stage of my career) and I'm telling you I wouldn't go near your dog unless he had a muzzle on. Do you have a muzzle for him?"

"No," the son admitted. I had been rough with him and I could see the resentment starting to build. So I turned quickly to the mother, who was watching with some satisfaction, believing I was clearly on her side of the conflict. "Have you helped your son find a trainer for the dog?" I asked.

She replied, "No, I don't know anything about training dogs. And besides, he doesn't want any help."

"Well, he needs help, and lots of it. Have you offered to help your son with the expense of building a proper exercise pen or with fencing in your yard, so the dog has a safe place to play?" It was the son's turn to feel vindicated. I felt certain this was not the first time these issues had been discussed.

To me, the course of action seemed perfectly clear and obvious. First, the son had to recognize that he owned a dangerous, untrained dog that could not be let loose in public and must be safely confined. Next, the mother had to realize that this dog represented far more than just a dog. It was tied in with the loss of a father; for her son, losing the dog would be like losing his father all over again. To avoid alienating her son, she had to try to help him with this problem dog.

Yes, it all seemed clear and simple to me at 7:30 p.m. It seemed less simple at 8:30 and even less so at 9:30. When I finally walked out of the hospital with them at 11:30 p.m. that night, I was completely exhausted. After four hours of arguing, accusing, cajoling, and reasoning, several things were agreed upon, and I typed them out, gave each person a copy, and kept one for the medical record:

The son agreed his dog must have training and could not be let loose in public. It was to be either on a leash or behind a proper, eight-foot high fence—not tied out on a chain. This was to happen within the next four days, or else the dog had to be put in a boarding kennel until suitable restraint was provided.

If the dog attacked another person, bite wound or not, it was to be put to sleep.

The mother was to help locate and employ a competent trainer to help with the aggressive behavior. When it was safe for her to do so, she was to participate

S T E V E N   B .   M E T Z ,   D . V . M .

in that training.

The mother was to help financially with the building of a proper exercise area for the dog, and help with his care and feeding when it was safe for her to do so.

I cannot say that either of them seemed thrilled with these agreements but I hoped that at least the son would not be leaving home, and the dog would be prevented from attacking anyone else. I made sure they paid the cost of an emergency office call: $32.50 at that time. Not exactly the cost of four hours of family counseling by a trained psychologist!

That was my first night on call at the Warwick Animal Hospital. Not all on-call nights were like this. Some were more like the set of a war movie, featuring pets with wounds of all descriptions; others found dogs that had lost arguments with porcupines; or had eaten rubber toys, articles of clothing, or silverware (including knives); and some on-call nights simply had pets with sore skin, ears, or legs.

One such evening involved a large black Labrador retriever who had been struck by a car. He came in groaning in pain but able to walk on all four legs. When I looked at his gums and tongue, they were white instead of the normal pink, which indicated either circulatory shock or blood loss or both. When I felt his abdomen, he again groaned; the abdomen was distended and felt full. I had not been a veterinary practitioner very long, but given the history of having been hit by a car, pale gums and tongue, and a painful, fluid-feeling abdomen, the diagnosis was not difficult. This dog was almost certainly bleeding internally, and if we didn't stop the bleeding quickly we would lose this patient.

I thought about single-handedly attempting what would probably turn out to be a long and difficult surgery. My task would be to first start a blood transfusion to replace some of the blood the dog had already lost and was continuing to lose. Then I would need to quickly and safely anesthetize this already dangerously compromised patient, remove the blood filling the abdomen, locate the source of the bleeding, and stop that bleeding somehow. My mind was racing, *I'm never going to be able to do this quickly enough or expertly enough to save this dog's life.* Speed in surgery comes primarily with experience—experience I did not yet have.

Just as I was about to give the owners—a young couple who obviously adored their dog—a poor prognosis, in walked Dr. Maurice. He had just come from attending a cocktail party and stopped in to see how the youngest, least experienced of his professional staff was faring through a night on call. He was dressed in a suit and tie, a white, starched shirt, and well-polished shoes. It was a startling flashback to that moment when Dr. Fred Sattler walked through the door of the Southeast Alaska Veterinary Clinic just when I needed help with Henry, the mule with tetanus. Every time I was in a tight spot, it seemed, along came the cavalry to the rescue.

I outlined the situation to Dr. Maurice. He asked two questions, "Have you explained the problem and the risks to the owners, and told them the likely possibility of an unhappy ending? And are you prepared for a difficult rest of the evening?" When the young couple pleaded with me to do everything possible to save their beloved dog, I told Dr. Maurice that I was ready. Without further word, he peeled off his coat, tie, and white shirt, and we took the dog to surgery. For over an hour, Dr. Maurice (with my relatively inexperienced help) tried to repair the damage to the abdominal blood vessels caused by the impact of the automobile. The injuries were so severe that in spite of all our efforts, including administering two units of blood, we could not save the poor dog. Both Dr. Maurice and I were exhausted afterward, but the appreciation from the owners was more reward than any monetary fee.

From this case, I learned yet another important lesson. Though Dr. Maurice recognized the probable sad outcome, he didn't hesitate—the owners had left no doubt they wanted us to try to save their companion. Likewise, once we began the surgery, there were no half measures. We tried everything we knew to repair the damage. It was important for our professional self-respect to be able to look back and know we had done all that we could, and in so doing, earned the trust of our clients.

The most lethal "disease" we treated at Warwick—the number one killer— was the automobile. Leash laws were comparatively rare, and most people seemed to think nothing of letting their dogs and cats roam free, at night, including black dogs and cats on dark nights. The consequences were entirely predictable. What was not so predictable was the response of the owner when it came to treatment of the traumatized pet. Some owners were willing and eager to do everything possible to save a badly injured pet, no matter what the cost, like the young couple and their Labrador retriever. Others were quick to use the magic phrase, "Better put it to sleep, Doctor." Sometimes cost of treatment was the issue, sometimes it was the prospect of nursing the injured pet or living with an injured pet. Such decisions were often very painful for both owner and veterinarian.

The third category of owner required a type of outright cynicism familiar to any veterinary practitioner who has been in private practice a significant time. I refer to the owner who, when presented with the care options for the injured pet, responds, "Fix 'er up, Doc. I don't care what it costs." But they have either no intention or no means of paying for the care right from the beginning. It often requires the skill of a trained interrogator to discover this fact.

It was while on call I learned perhaps the most important lesson any veterinarian in private practice should learn: Never prejudge what decision a pet owner will make regarding the care of a patient. Always present all options and let the owner decide. On a typical evening while on call, at about midnight, two elderly ladies brought a calico cat to me. The cat had returned home after having been let out earlier that evening. The cat was dragging her hind legs, unable to bear weight on either one. The ladies were both dressed in housecoats— none too clean—and slippers. I happened to glance out into the parking lot and noticed that the car they were driving was also elderly. To complete the picture, their cat was twelve years old, the human equivalent of which is about sixty-five.

After examining the cat, I determined that the most likely cause for the unusable hind legs was either a fractured pelvis or a broken back. To find out, I would need to x-ray the cat under sedation to avoid causing pain or possibly worsening the injuries if the kitty were to struggle. I described all this to the two ladies and told them what the emergency examination, sedation, and x-rays would cost. I explained that neither of the two possible causes of injury boded well. A broken back meant it was extremely unlikely the cat would ever be able to walk again, while a broken pelvis might mean the same thing, or at least a prolonged recovery. In addition, the cat's ability to control her bladder or intestinal function might be impaired.

Many owners at this point would have opted for putting the kitty to sleep. The two ladies immediately requested that I proceed with the x-rays. These owners were not regular clients of the Warwick Animal Hospital, so I had no record of any previous financial transactions. As required by hospital policy, but feeling quite reluctant to bring up the subject, I reminded them they would be responsible for payment that night. They assured me they were prepared to take care of expenses. I thus sedated the cat carefully and took the required films, which showed a badly fractured pelvis.

Because the pelvis is a box-like structure providing its own braces, many times a fracture in one or even two places requires only rest to heal. This poor kitty had several fractures and the pelvis was quite unstable. Surgery would almost certainly be required for the cat to walk again. Pelvic surgery, even today, is considered major orthopedic surgery and none of the four other veterinarians at Warwick Animal Hospital were surgeon specialists. Even Dr. Maurice and Dr. Robbin, with all their experience, were not trained nor equipped to perform this type of surgery. It would require a specialist.

This presented two problems for these owners: No orthopedic surgeon specialists lived in the entire state of Rhode Island. The closest was at Angell Animal Medical Center in Boston, Massachusetts, about a two-hour drive away. Even in the 1970s, the services of specialist surgeons were costly, particularly for a surgery as involved as this would be. I anticipated the cost for the surgery and aftercare would approach $1,000—a staggering fee back then, though quite routine today. There was no pet insurance at that time. I discussed all this with the two elderly ladies in housecoats (who drove the elderly, dilapidated car), fully expecting to hear something like, "I suppose we must put her to sleep. She is twelve years old. We can't possibly drive to Boston. We can't afford the services of a specialist performing such a costly surgery."

Instead, to my complete astonishment, one of the ladies reached into the pocket of her housecoat and extracted a thick roll of bills. I had enough wit to notice that at least the top few bills were of $100 denomination.

"Will this do for a deposit?" she asked. "We have more at home and friends in Boston where we can stay while Kitty is recovering from her operation."

I was speechless. When I recovered, I stammered, "Would you like me to call the hospital in Boston and alert them you will be coming and your cat will need to see Dr. Robert Griffith, the orthopedic surgeon?" They agreed, and paid their bill in cash, all large bills. Controlling my sagging jaw, I helped them make Kitty comfortable in the back seat of their car. As they were getting ready to drive away, I heard one ask the other, "Are we going to stop at home for clothes and more money?" The one with the roll of bills in her pocket answered, "No, we can always buy what we need in Boston and we can call the bank and have them send us some money." And away they drove.

The next morning I received a call from Dr. Griffith, one of the most unassuming, generous, and skillful veterinary surgeons and colleagues I have encountered. He thanked me for referring the case to him (not all surgeons would have been entirely pleased by having such a difficult surgery referred to them, by the way) and then asked if I had discussed the cost of a pelvic fracture repair with the ladies. He added, "We can certainly make things as easy as possible for them, but just the materials and nursing staff will be quite costly, no matter what I write off." Even an experienced practitioner like Dr. Griffith was deceived by appearances; I didn't feel like such a fool. I couldn't resist telling Dr. Griffith my experience with these owners—including the "pocket change" I had seen the previous evening. He chuckled and said, "It's been a good lesson for both of us, hasn't it?"

I don't remember what the total bill for this case was, but I do remember that approximately three months later, the receptionist asked me to come to the waiting room; two elderly ladies wanted to show me a cat. The nurse finished by saying, "Remember, Dr. Metz, we must charge for our services." The minute I saw these two ladies I recognized them. "How did your Kitty do?" I asked, half-dreading the answer. In response, they opened up one of two wicker baskets they had carried in. A sleek, elderly cat jumped out of the basket and walked around the reception area. Barely a trace of a wobble remained in the hind legs! What a testament to the skill of Dr. Robert Griffith, the recuperative powers of cats, and the power of the owners' devotion to their companion.

Before I had a chance to say anything else, one of the ladies presented me with the other wicker basket. "Thank you for all your help, Dr. Metz." They gathered up Kitty and left, still driving the old car. When I opened the wicker basket, my eyes popped: It was full of gourmet food, including caviar and a small bottle of very expensive champagne. Moments like these are to be cherished, because in addition to the champagne and caviar, it happens all too frequently that you find yourself powerless to help someone's beloved pet in distress.

I had been at the Warwick Animal Hospital almost a year when we received an unusual call. The supervisor of animal care at the Roger Williams Park Zoo, just two miles up the road from our hospital, was asking for help. A full-grown male ostrich had poked his head through an opening in a wire fence and cut his eyelid. The supervisor asked if one of our doctors could come to the zoo and suture the cut. Three of us were in the hospital at the time, and I was the junior doctor. Dr. Robbin was just about to go into surgery, and Dr. Seidler had absolutely no enthusiasm for working with a large ostrich. I volunteered immediately. The prospect of working with exotic and unusual animals filled me with excitement. To me this was one of the most stimulating and rewarding parts of our great profession.

I packed everything I could think of into our veterinary traveling bags. One problem was restraint; ostriches are huge, powerful birds, distrustful of humans. They almost always resent any handling, especially around their head and eyes. Their usual way of demonstrating resentment is to deliver lightning-fast kicks with their powerful legs, the toes of which are equipped with strong, sharp toenails. Ostriches are quite capable of causing severe injury to anyone around them. Because I would be suturing very close to the eye, I would need the head to be absolutely still.

Avian medicine was still in its infancy at this time; treatment of large flightless birds such as ostriches, emus, and cassowaries—members of the ratite family—was an adventure into the unknown. As far as I knew, there was no accepted method or medication for anesthetizing these animals. A few reports on hawks mentioned ketamine, a relatively new injectable compound being used mostly in primates and children. But even the largest hawk differs greatly in size and metabolic rate from an ostrich. As any veterinarian knows, medication given to one species versus another species can result in very different reactions. I wondered whether ketamine would be safe and effective for anesthetizing an ostrich, and where I should inject it, and how much I should use. I had never been up close and personal with an ostrich and certainly had never operated on one.

Here, however, was the wonder of a veterinary education. I knew that, with few exceptions, skin is skin—and the principles of wound repair in one species generally hold true for most other species (until you come to specially modified skin, such as that of reptiles). This same education and these same principles enabled me to treat such diverse patients as a tiger with hepatitis, an elephant with pink eye, and a fish with fin rot.

I arrived at the Roger Williams Park Zoo where the keeper responsible for the bird section was waiting. I expect he had some doubts when he saw a new face instead of Dr. Maurice or Dr. Robbin, and even more doubts when I told him I planned to use a new drug on his ostrich. "Mighty expensive bird to use for an experiment," was his dubious comment. He would have preferred good old-fashioned manual restraint—euphemistically called Brutacaine by some veterinarians—and he had several husky zoo helpers ready to wrestle the ostrich to a standstill. I explained that suturing around the eye during a struggle would not be safe for the bird or for people.

We built a wall of hay bales around the tall male ostrich so he couldn't kick. With the expert help of the keeper I administered a conservative dose of ketamine in the large drumstick muscle. Then we all stood back and watched. In about five minutes, the big fellow became unsteady on his legs and with the help of the keeper, we persuaded him to sit down. His small head remained wiggly on top of his four-foot long neck. As the keeper stood on a hay bale and

Steven B. Metz, d.v.m.

grasped the ostrich's neck just below the head to steady it, I climbed on top of two hay bales to reach the eye area. The cut was right at the outside corner of the left eye. Considerable care was required to align the edges accurately, so the patient would end up with properly shaped eyelids that would protect the eye as they were supposed to. The stitching took several minutes, because I had to time each stitch to when the keeper was able to keep the head absolutely still. Considering the problems we would have removing these sutures, I used a non-reactive nylon material and cut the knots short, so the stitches could be left in. For all I know, that ostrich went to his grave wearing those stitches; I, for one, wasn't going to try to remove them.

That may well have been the first time ketamine was used in a member of the ostrich family. I felt a sense of accomplishment at being able to suture a tricky area on an animal notoriously difficult to handle. And no humans were injured. Had I been more academically inclined, I think I could have published a paper on the case in our professional Journal of the American Veterinary Medical Association. I had been out of school only about a year, however, and the idea of someone so new to the practice of veterinary medicine breaking new ground was difficult for me to accept. I still saw myself a student, especially compared to my mentors Dr. Maurice and Dr. Robbin. But from that time on, the personnel at the Roger Williams Park Zoo asked for me when they encountered a problem.

I experienced one other remarkable visit to the zoo that closely mirrors something Dr. J.Y. Henderson described in his book, Circus Doctor. The zoo had a small collection of large cats that included a male leopard. He was housed in a spacious enclosure and his keeper reported that he was very friendly. He loved to have his neck scratched and would come to the fence for a neck-scratching session every morning. A few days before, the keeper had noticed a bump on the leopard's chin and thought it might be an abscess. I looked at the spot through the fence and agreed with the keeper's diagnosis. I suggested he try to get the leopard to tolerate warm compresses on the chin to see if we could localize the infection. I had a hazy idea of somehow opening and draining it, as is the usual treatment of an abscess, although I had no idea how I would get the leopard to agree to this treatment. This keeper was sure he could make a game of the compresses. The plan was for me to come back several days later to see how the area looked.

In my experience, people working in legitimate organizations or establishments, who are responsible for the care and management of wild or non-domestic animals, including marine species, are an extraordinarily dedicated group. Many are unpaid or minimally paid volunteers who donate their time and efforts out of love and respect for the animals. I have personally observed the real affection and concern keepers and trainers have for the wellbeing of their charges. There are exceptions, mostly at so-called wild animal farms, or commercial exhibits where financial gain is the primary objective and where inspection or regulation is minimal.

At times animal keepers and trainers risk their own safety to provide care for animals that do not appreciate their caregiving efforts, contrary to the often-voiced and mistaken opinion that animals "know you're trying to help them." We commonly hear of keepers injured by animals they have cared for years. I believe that when these injuries or accidents occur it is because the keeper or trainer becomes careless or forgets that the animal being cared for is first, last, and always, a wild creature whose world is governed by a totally different set of instincts and environmental responses than our own.

So as I prepared to deal with the leopard abscess at the Roger Williams Park Zoo, I recalled a day when I stood wide-eyed beside Dr. J.Y. Henderson at Ringling Brothers Circus. We were listening to one of the big cat trainers discuss this very same subject. The trainer told the story (also narrated in Dr. Henderson's book) of his years working in his circus act with one particular female leopard named Sonya. At the end of his mixed act (lions, tigers, and leopards all in the same ring together), he would drive all the other cats out of the ring except Sonya. Then he would drop his chair and the bamboo sticks that he used to signal and prod his performers during the act. He would hold out his arms to Sonya; she would drop from her pedestal, walk to him, stand on her hind legs, and put her head on his shoulder. He would then put his arm around her and the two of them would walk out of the ring together. What a spectacular finale!

The trainer's purpose in telling this story was to note that in spite of having performed this finale over and over again with Sonya, he knew there were times she was more nervous or upset. He said, "If you watch me closely you will see that when I feel Sonya is upset I tuck my chin and head into my shoulder, so if she should attack me, I might have a chance to fight back." I remember the chill running through me, as I thought of Sonya, as sweet as a house kitten, attacking and mauling the trainer who fed her, groomed her, and took care of her for so many years. Stories like this one make me skeptical when I hear of wild creatures described as tame or friendly—just the way the keeper at the Roger Williams Park Zoo was describing his male leopard.

S t e v e n   B .   M e t z ,   d . v . m .

I was therefore determined not to do anything outright silly or dangerous in dealing with the abscess on the leopard's chin. When I arrived at the leopard's enclosure with the keeper, I was carrying a small, very sharp scalpel blade in my hand. The big male leopard, impressive when viewed up close, came to the fence to be scratched. Predictably, the cage bars were just a bit too narrow to fit my hand and wrist through with any reasonable maneuverability.

"How have you been applying the warm compresses twice daily?" I asked the leopard's keeper.

"Oh, I just went into the enclosure with him, and we made sort of a game of it," he replied. He unlocked the gate, stepped into the enclosure, and began scratching the leopard under the chin, looking at me expectantly.

I really did not want to go into an enclosure with an unsedated adult leopard. But the abscess, or "furuncle," on the big male's chin was much too minor to justify giving him a general anesthetic. My choice was either to refuse to treat the patient or to walk into that enclosure. I felt if I refused to walk into the enclosure, I would lose the respect of the personnel at the Roger Williams Park Zoo. But I couldn't be sure this fellow would even accept me putting a hand on him!

"Bring him over to the bars," I directed the keeper, hoping I could figure out a way—from outside the enclosure—of opening the furuncle so it would drain. When the keeper brought Mr. Leopard up to the bars, I hesitantly reached through and scratched the underside of his lower jaw, within easy reach of a mouthful of huge teeth. The big cat seemed to enjoy it. I, meanwhile, was not enjoying it, because I knew that it would only take one minute and I might well be minus a hand.

Try as I might, I could not twist my wrist and hand into position to lance the abscess through the bars. So reluctantly, and calling myself a total fool, I walked into the enclosure. I told the keeper to keep scratching—don't stop. Taking a deep breath, I gave the leopard's chin two scratches, reversed my hand, and with the scalpel blade I was carrying between my fingers, I pierced the abscess.

The big fellow jerked his head and stepped back a few paces, and I did exactly the same thing. In one motion, and seemingly without any direction from me, my legs went automatically into reverse. I was out the door, and calling the keeper to come out as I went. He did not follow me. To this day, I carry a picture in my mind's eye of that large male leopard rubbing his head against his keeper's thigh as a small amount of blood-tinged discharge dripped from his chin.

"Pretty slick, Doc!" called the keeper; he had to raise his voice because I was already most of the way to my car in the parking lot. Pretty damn stupid, I said to myself. I'll never do anything like that again! Naturally, this resolution was not to last.

My practical education continued. Each day brought new challenges, new learning opportunities—sometimes heartbreak, sometimes rich rewards. I began to feel more confident when I walked into an examination room that I would be able to help the companion pet and their owner, or at least point them in a helpful direction if a problem was beyond my capabilities. For this too is a critical part of any doctor's education: to learn your limitations and recognize the moment when another opinion or another approach is best for the patient or for the owner.

As I began my third year as an associate veterinary practitioner at the Warwick Animal Hospital, certain questions about the future direction of my career and my family started to gain more importance. We were by then a family of five, having recently welcomed our son Jamie into the world; he arrived in a rather exciting way.

On the evening of September 13, 1972 at approximately 8 p.m., Connie felt some stirrings that led us to believe Jamie's arrival was imminent. As it happened, our route to Connie's hospital took us right past the Warwick Animal Hospital, and as we got closer to it, Connie said, "I can't wait till Providence, pull into the veterinary hospital and you'll have to deliver the baby!"

By this time in my career, I had delivered many puppies and kittens, and I had done several Caesarian section surgeries. You might think I would be somewhat prepared for such an event. Instead, I was seized by such terror at the prospect of having to deliver my own child that I shouted, "No! No! Wait!" I wrenched the steering wheel to the left, drove right across the grass median of the interstate, and headed straight for the small county hospital in East Greenwich only a few miles away. All this time, Connie was urging me to pull over.

When I drove into the emergency room parking lot, I was dismayed to see a flight of stairs at the entrance of the hospital. Connie certainly couldn't navigate them in her present condition. Without thinking about how much my pregnant wife might weigh, I scooped her up in my arms and ran up the steps. I burst into the emergency room where two nurses sat chatting. "Quick!" I gasped. "She's having a baby right now!" To their credit, the nurses asked no questions and wheeled a stretcher right up to me, and I laid Connie on it. One nurse wheeled Connie to the elevator and I followed. The other nurse phoned the delivery room to get ready for a "quickie"—I actually heard her use that term. But as ready as they might have been, our son had done all the waiting he was going to do. He entered the world on that stretcher on the way to the delivery room. Connie didn't even get her coat off, and the nurses didn't get to put on their gloves. I was left standing in the hall while the whole procedure was completed. Approximately fifteen minutes later, Connie and I were in a hospital room staring at each other. "What happened?" we both asked simultaneously. A few hours after that, we were on our way home with our new addition.

Medicine is entirely different when it involves "your own." This is as valid for pets as it is for children, spouses, or other family members. Certainly, I could have given my wife the necessary immediate assistance (not that any was needed, as it turned out) until we arrived at a suitable hospital, but I was panic-stricken. Never mind that I had managed much more complicated births at the Warwick Animal Hospital. This was different; this was my own family.

This is an important lesson for the companion animal veterinary practitioner because of how often we are asked by pet owners if they can watch while their pet has surgery. The owners assure us that nothing bothers them. I learned early in my career to be skeptical of such requests, and of owners who are insistent on viewing their pet's surgery. I require that they watch surgery on someone else's companion first. I also impress upon them that my first responsibility is to the patient, and I can only treat one patient at a time. As hard as I try, I sometimes get fooled and my technicians end up caring for an owner who suddenly feels faint. Often this happens to a person I would least expect to have difficulty. Under the right circumstances I agree to an owner watching surgery on their pet, because it can be a marvelous opportunity to educate the pet-owning public about the value of modern veterinary medicine and to demonstrate the skill and training of the person they've chosen to care for their companion.

The lessons I was learning about the art of practice as well as the science of veterinary medicine caused me to seek input into management decisions at the Warwick Animal Hospital. Although I had been an associate for over two years, I had little role in policy decisions. It would be only as a partner that I would have the right and the responsibility of decision-making. Looking back, it seems presumptuous of me to expect to have earned a partnership after only two years. Still, I felt compelled to at least discuss the subject with Dr. Maurice and Dr. Robbin. They listened carefully to my request, and then answered in the forthright manner for which I had such great respect. Both doctors had younger children who might want a career in veterinary medicine; they would deserve the chance to assume ownership. Besides, these two veterinarians had spent more than fifteen years building the practice, and intended to take great care before handing over any part of the decision-making to anyone else.

So no prospect of part ownership existed for me in the foreseeable future. This was disappointing because I had such respect and affection for both doctors; I was sure that if I were willing to be a long-term employee of anyone, it would have been for them. Both doctors assured me if I remained at Warwick, I could expect a significant increase in salary.

It was a dilemma: to stay in a busy, challenging practice and enjoy almost certain financial security, or look for another practice where there was a chance of becoming a partner. The idea of striking out on my own and starting a brand new practice seemed quite out of reach. I felt I didn't have the experience or the professional skill required to manage my own practice only two years out of school, to say nothing of the financial wherewithal to purchase an existing practice, or to build a practice from scratch.

This was obviously a family decision, perhaps more vital to our future than our decision to join the staff of the Warwick Animal Hospital. We had to decide where to look for a practice and whether or not to stay in Rhode Island. We had to revisit our original decision to stay in New England—or at least the Northeast—to test if it still reflected our feelings almost three years later. In 1972, without the Internet, it was going to be a challenge to find the sort of opportunity I was looking for. Nonetheless, I soon began the search for what I hoped would be our final destination.

Steven B. Metz, d.v.m.

chapter six

The Ultimate Gamble

The first decision Connie and I made was to stay in New England if at all possible. I found myself wishing for a less crowded, more rural setting to bring up our children. I wanted to become a contributing member of a community and to develop friendships with neighbors. As we have seen, veterinary medicine sometimes involves intervening as if a family counselor. A pet owner ought to know the person to whom they turn for help, and the more familiar with family dynamics and circumstances a veterinary practitioner is, the more appropriate the advice and help they can offer.

With this lifestyle in mind, we agreed to look for opportunities in northern New England: Maine, New Hampshire, and Vermont. I spent every spare weekend driving around northern New England to locate existing veterinary practices, gauge the potential for a new veterinary practice, and trying to get a sense of what the various communities had to offer. Some of these weekends were spent in our little Volkswagen, bumping over backcountry roads, asking unexpected questions of complete strangers, and meeting local veterinarians who were left wondering whether they were about to be invaded. I took my father along on one such weekend jaunt. He was completely unused to being in such a small vehicle, and later told me that after that time spent in the Bug, he felt his insides had been rearranged.

During this time of exploration, I answered two professional advertisements in the Journal of the American Veterinary Medical Association: one in Portland, Maine and the other in Rutland, Vermont. The opportunity in Portland turned out to have no prospects for partnership, and a startling coincidence occurred at the Eastwind Animal Hospital just outside Rutland. Initially, I spoke with the practice owner Dr. Blair Campbell. He showed me around his attractive modern hospital, and we had an agreeable talk. The result was that Dr. Campbell offered me a position as associate veterinarian, and that if we were personally and professionally compatible after a trial period of one year, I would be able to begin purchasing ownership of the practice by stages. Dr.

Campbell promised to send me the written contract containing the points we had agreed upon. It was late October 1972, and I left Rutland feeling I was well on my way to realizing my goal of practice ownership.

By the end of November, I still had not received the promised contract. When I called Dr. Campbell, he said there had been a delay in getting the papers drawn up, but I would be hearing from him soon. Meanwhile, to be fair to Drs. Maurice and Robbin, I told them I was planning to leave, even though I didn't yet have a firm date. They made sure I knew I was welcome to stay at Warwick if I couldn't find a suitable situation. Connie and I felt quite unsettled and unable to make some important decisions because I had no definite commitment.

On Christmas Eve, I received a phone call from Dr. Campbell. He said he had some bad news for me. A veterinary classmate of his with whom he had been particularly friendly had called Dr. Campbell and asked if he could have the position. This classmate explained that he had had a terrible argument with the primary practice owner and he needed to leave right away. Dr. Campbell said he really had no choice; he felt he must give the position to his classmate.

The unfortunate coincidence was that this classmate was none other than Dr. Ingram—the veterinarian who had so impressed me at the Riverhead, Long Island practice three years before as I was on my whirlwind interview tour of twenty-one practices. I might have ended up in Riverhead because of Dr. Ingram, and now I had lost out on a position because of him. Of course, Dr. Campbell had the right to employ whomever he pleased. I particularly understood the choice of Dr. Ingram, a friend and known quantity. Unfortunately, this all left me completely without a prospect for joining either practice.

I continued my explorations. After my experiences trying to negotiate partnership within existing practices, I was beginning to feel that my best option was to open my own practice. My final decision was made after a conversation with the newest veterinary member of the staff at Warwick, Dr. Fred Karotkin. One day, as we discussed the desirability of opening a new practice, he asked me simply, "What are you afraid of?" And when I tried to answer, I realized I had nothing to fear. My education and training had been excellent all the way along. Now when I stepped into an examination room or took a patient into surgery, I had some experience. I could picture exactly what I would do differently from the way things were managed at Warwick. I wanted a small, personalized practice, where I would see every patient and every family.

There are advantages and disadvantages to each type of practice, of course.

With a difficult case at Warwick, there was always a colleague with whom the case could be discussed. Yet pet owners often saw different doctors each time they came for their appointment. I was ready to try the other extreme—solo practice. I just needed to find an area that would be most in need of a new, progressive companion animal hospital.

After many weekends spent scouting, I was attracted to Burlington, Vermont, on the shores of Lake Champlain. The medical school at the University of Vermont in Burlington was the only one of its caliber outside of Boston in all of New England, and provided a robust and compelling medical community. Three veterinary hospitals served the Burlington/South Burlington area and one practice was about a fifteen-minute drive away in Essex Junction. This seemed like a lot of veterinarians for the area's population. I paid a visit to all four area practices, introducing myself as being interested in starting a practice somewhere in the area. The reception I received at each practice was quite distinct and served to predict, quite accurately, my future relationships with these prospective colleagues.

Two veterinarians, Dr. Fred Aliesky of Aliesky Animal Hospital and Dr. Jon Stokes of the Green Mountain Animal Hospital, were welcoming and encouraging. Unfortunately, at the most established practice, the owner received me as if I were an unwelcome salesman; he was obviously unenthusiastic about a new practice or a new colleague. The fourth practice, Burlington Animal Hospital, was owned by Dr. Richard Fournier, a veterinarian with significant health problems. Because of these health problems, he felt it necessary to go to Florida for a month or more during the winter. When I asked him if he thought the area could support another practice, he said gloomily, "There's barely enough work for the practices already here." However, while I was in his hospital, two or three phone calls came from owners wanting appointments. Dr. Fournier put them all off, using telephone advice rather than examining the pet. Perhaps I was being judgmental, but at the Warwick Animal Hospital, those patients would have been seen. Dr. Fournier was not realizing the full earning potential of his practice. I asked him if he would consider taking on an associate, but he repeated that his practice would not support another veterinarian. I then asked him if he had ever considered selling his practice. He replied that he was not ready to sell just yet.

I felt frustrated. Here we had a practitioner who was in ill health, obviously did not want to grow his practice, but at the same time, he was complaining that the practice was not profitable. He didn't want to employ another practitioner (who would not have to take a month or two off), and he didn't want to sell this unprofitable practice. This was a pity because his practice was located on U.S. Route 7, one of two major routes into Burlington. It was the busiest highway in the state at the time. No other practices were between his hospital and the small city of Vergennes, some twenty-five minutes south—and that practice was owned by a veterinarian who had far more experience with farm animals than companion pets.

After much exploration and soul-searching, and many family conferences with my parents, my neurologist older brother, my wife's parents, and my revered grandfather, I decided to take the plunge and start a practice in the small town of Shelburne, Vermont, just seven miles south of Burlington. I knew absolutely no one, and we did not have a place to live. Also, I had yet to obtain financing for purchasing the necessary property and building and equipping from scratch a modern, attractive, functional veterinary hospital. I was barely three years out of veterinary college, and I had accumulated no great savings. I located a wonderful property in Shelburne, right on U.S. Route 7, and my next step was to visit the three main area banks to obtain a loan. All this time I was still working full-time at Warwick, a seven-hour drive away.

Arming myself with facts and figures about real estate expenses, the cost of building a veterinary hospital, and the profitability of a well-run companion animal veterinary practice, I met with loan officers from each bank. What an education I received! Each loan officer's response to my proposal and request for financial help was startlingly different.

The first banker with whom I spoke listened with a tolerant smile, and when I finished, he said, "Dr. Metz, why don't you come back to see me when you have more information about your proposal." I felt as if he had patted me on the head and said, "Run along now, sonny, and come back when you're older." Bank officer number two listened, and said, "It sounds encouraging, and I'm sure we can work things out. Here's my card. Call when you know exactly what you'll need." I had one financial authority dismissing my plan to open a new veterinary practice as incomplete and inadequately thought out, while another loan officer in the same city was eager to help. I was completely confused! Was my plan sensible or not?

I went to the third bank and spoke with Stephen Moore. He listened carefully to the information I presented without changing his expression and without any comments or questions. I remember thinking to myself, Boy, this is one tough fellow. I wonder how fast he'll show me to the door? When I finished,

Steven B. Metz, d.v.m.

Mr. Moore sat back in his chair, gave me a small grin, and said, "You are talking to probably the only banker in the entire state of Vermont who has a daughter in veterinary college … big advantage, Dr. Metz." And sure enough, so it proved to be. With moral and financial support from several family members, and with the guidance of Stephen Moore, the Shelburne Veterinary Hospital became a possibility, but not yet a reality. My next step was to find the right builder.

I picked three medium-sized contractors out of the yellow pages. Once I had made the decision to leave Warwick Animal Hospital I began visiting other veterinary hospitals to get ideas for my own building. I found stark contrasts in veterinary hospital design, materials used, and equipment. I took extensive notes during these hospital visits, and often discussed my observations and questions with Dr. Maurice and Dr. Robbin, both of whom were generous with suggestions and advice. I ended up writing a set of specifications detailing what materials were to be used in each part of the hospital, what size each room needed to be, what type of heating, air-conditioning, and ventilation systems should be installed, what capacity electrical system, what type of plumbing, and specific notes about flooring.

In 1972, veterinary hospital construction was largely experimental. All sorts of designs and materials were used on a trial-and-error basis; there was no standard. An architect's idea of a veterinary hospital could be almost anything. All this would change with the emergence of standards set by the American Animal Hospital Association (AAHA). This group had developed a set of standards for hospital design, management, and methods of medical and surgical veterinary practice with the goal of encouraging excellence in companion animal practice. To become a member hospital, you had to meet demanding requirements involving every aspect of hospital management and practice— from how the floors were cleaned and how many changes of air occurred in the building per hour to what methods of anesthesia and surgery were employed. A hospital applying for certification had to undergo a thorough inspection, which took almost a whole day. Being an AAHA-certified member hospital showed that the owner placed major emphasis in achieving excellence in the practice of veterinary medicine.

I was determined right from the start that my hospital would qualify as an AAHA-member hospital. I consulted with the AAHA home office frequently as I drew up plans for the design and construction of the Shelburne Veterinary Hospital. In my naiveté, I thought all I had to do was find a builder who would carefully follow the specifications I had written. I was to have yet another learning experience, this time about building contractors and the building process.

The first construction firm I approached asked, "Where are the architectural drawings, the blueprints?" I explained I was not using an architect because of the unusual requirements of the building. He answered, "We cannot possibly construct a building without an architect being involved. We don't handle design and construction. Sorry we cannot be of help at this time." The second firm did have a design department, but could not undertake the project for several months, and warned me they could not make a final decision as to whether this project was something they felt they could bid on until they had seen the proposed blueprints. In this case, it was possible I could pay the company for an architect's services but still not have a willing contractor. Not to mention, I was hoping to get started right away so that I could end my term at Warwick and move our family.

My third try was the charm—as it had been with the bank financing. I met with Mr. Frank Alling of the Alling Construction Company. No departments, no specialists, no consultants. Just Frank Alling—the good-natured, easygoing owner of his company. At our first meeting, when I told him I wanted to build a veterinary hospital, he said, "That ought to be easy. We can just convert a barn." I gently explained this was to be a companion animal hospital with a surgery room, x-ray area, laboratory, pharmacy, treatment and recovery area, examination rooms, indoor kennels, and a reception area. Each room had its own requirements for design and materials. For example, the surgery room needed an extra-high ceiling to allow mounted overhead surgical lights, a one-way air flow to prevent dust or germs from getting into the room, special paint to enhance the lighting and visibility, and special acid-washed copper tubing to carry oxygen from outside—not only to the surgery room but to several different areas of the hospital.

Frank Alling's expression became more and more thoughtful. Next I handed him the twenty-five pages of specifications and said, "I don't have an architect or blueprints." I waited, half expecting to hear that he couldn't proceed without an architect, as the other two firms had told me. Instead, Frank's response was, "No problem, I can do any drawings or blueprints we need. An architect would probably get in the way, anyhow."

As he scanned my notes, he started nodding: he knew just the kind of material required, he knew just the person who could install the type of flooring I wanted, and so on.

His eyebrows raised a notch when he read I would need at least ten tons of

Steven B. Metz, d.v.m.

air-conditioning capacity. He protested, "This is Vermont. You don't need air conditioning." I explained it in this way: "Picture my examination room, Frank. In the room is a big, panting, slobbery Saint Bernard with a fever of 103. Also in the room is the owner, who is anxious about her sick doggie, and she has brought her three children, who are running back and forth checking out all the instruments and cupboards in the room. What do you think the temperature in that examination room will reach?" He understood and that was the last time he questioned the necessity of any of my specifications.

Best of all, Frank said he could get started almost immediately, work through the winter, and have the building finished by spring of 1973. Thus began my great adventure: the creation of a brand new and very modern veterinary hospital. I was to become an owner and an employer. Success or failure of this enterprise would rest entirely on my judgment, hard work, and professional skill. As much as it is possible in life to be in charge of your own destiny, this seemed to be my time and place.

I would have to learn to make many decisions purely from a business standpoint—nothing to do with veterinary medicine. I must now develop people skills to attract and develop a following of new clients. Although I might become a technically skillful veterinary practitioner, all would be meaningless unless I could communicate successfully with the owner of the patient. The future of my new practice and the wellbeing of our family depended on these skills.

One major obstacle to the construction of the Shelburne Veterinary Hospital remained; I needed a permit from the Town of Shelburne Zoning Board and Planning Commission. Without the approval of these authorities, no building could take place. The residents of Shelburne were quite determined to maintain the flavor of a small, elegant residential community and to avoid allowing U.S. Route 7, known as Shelburne Road, to become a strip mall. Directly behind my proposed hospital was a small residential development. My hospital would directly adjoin its backyards. What would happen if these prospective neighbors showed up at the zoning board hearing and protested a veterinary hospital next to their peaceful homes? After all, who would want barking dogs right next to their yards? There might be odors associated with a veterinary hospital, or the building might be unattractive. Other neighbors might have no specific complaint about a veterinary hospital, but might wish to keep the land free of further development for aesthetic reasons. The Shelburne Zoning Board had a reputation for being sharply critical when it came to commercial development. I realized a strong protest might influence them to deny a construction permit.

I gathered up the drawings and plans made by Frank Alling, and I began visiting door-to-door with my neighbors (and possible future clients); I went over all the details of the construction and operation of the Shelburne Veterinary Hospital. I took careful note of any concerns expressed, and made sure to return within twenty-four hours with a solution. The most common concern I heard was the potential for noise. If I were to have outdoor dog runs, barking was inevitable. I therefore completely eliminated all outdoor runs and altered the design to be as soundproof as possible. I further assured neighbors that I was a tree lover and would leave a substantial tree belt between the hospital and their yards. The building design was to be a combination of natural-stained wood and brick; it was a single story to minimize any impact on the view—as well as to save wear and tear on the doctor's knees.

The neighbors' response to my involving them in my building and operating plans was more favorable than I had hoped. On the evening of the zoning board hearing, a much larger than usual group was present. I noticed almost every person to whom I'd spoken. I hoped for the best, but I was apprehensive; my future was dependent on a favorable ruling and the issuance of a construction permit. When my name was called, I stood before the zoning board members. I had submitted the drawings and plans almost a month earlier and reviewed the construction plans. I emphasized that there would be no outdoor kennels, and soundproofing would be incorporated throughout the building. When I finished my presentation, the chair of the zoning board asked the audience if there were any comments or questions for Dr. Metz. One of the neighbors who had seemed the most concerned about having a veterinary hospital in his backyard raised his hand. I braced myself.

"Mr. Chairman, I've been asked to speak for the residents whose properties abut the proposed construction of a veterinary hospital. Dr. Metz has taken great care to address our concerns. We not only have no objection, but we feel this well-designed building and veterinary service will be a valuable addition to our area and to the town of Shelburne. We urge you to act favorably on this application." Never in my wildest dreams had I imagined such a response, especially from this man. In the end, with a few minor questions about landscaping, the Shelburne zoning board issued the permit.

So began the construction of the Shelburne Veterinary Hospital, my professional home for the next thirty-seven years. It is difficult to describe my feelings as I watched the building take shape. It was something akin to experiencing the birth of a child. Even the digging of the foundation was exciting. It is one thing

STEVEN B. METZ, D.V.M.

to look at blueprints and drawings, but there is no substitute for standing inside a room you have designed.

I had arranged with Drs. Maurice and Robbin that I would continue to work on Friday evenings, Saturdays, and Sundays. I would then climb in my car on Sunday evening and drive seven hours to Shelburne, so I could be on hand to oversee the construction and be available for any decisions—thus preventing any interruption in progress. Often during those drives, I would have to pull over for a short nap to avoid falling asleep at the wheel. Other times, I would arrive back in Shelburne an hour or two before the construction crew; on these occasions, I would park right by the building and try to nap. In 1972, Shelburne Road was not as developed as it is today; several mornings as the sun rose, I would watch a small group of deer come down the hill from behind the houses next to my property, trot across the highway, and go down to the shore of Lake Champlain.

I spent all week—from Monday morning until Thursday afternoon—helping coordinate schedules of the various subcontractors. The electricians couldn't begin until the framing and siding were done, and the plumbers couldn't do their job until the electricians were finished. Materials had to be purchased and payments made; it was a busy time. Then, suddenly, it got much busier. Frank Alling became involved in a lawsuit that almost completely prevented him from overseeing the construction. Thus, by default I became the general contractor. A few weeks later, the construction foreman, a huge man appropriately called Moose, fell and broke his hip. I thus became construction foreman, a position for which my only qualification was a thorough knowledge of the end product.

Fortunately, by spring of 1973 the building was more than halfway finished, the weather was turning warmer, and instead of frozen ground and frozen fingers, we had mud. All these months, I had been staying in a small, inexpensive motel just two miles from the construction. Now the time had come for two more steps that would complete the transition to practice owner. First, the Metz family had to find a place to live. In our eleven years of marriage, Connie and I had never owned a home. We had moved four times, and the longest we had stayed in one place was our four years in Eden Mills, Ontario. Soon there would be no more moves for the foreseeable future. I was a property owner, soon to be a practice owner—no more moves. The greater Burlington area was attractive with many fine places to live, but I had to be available twenty-four hours a day for emergencies. In fairness to my clients, I had to be able to respond to emergencies quickly, so finding a home relatively near the practice was important. We were fortunate to find a nice place in a small housing development two miles from the hospital. We would be residents of the town of Shelburne, which had the reputation for excellent schools. All three of our children would attend these schools and would receive a firm foundation for their continued education.

Now we had two mortgages. Could anyone have dug a deeper financial pit for themselves? All this debt without the guarantee of a single dollar of profit. To make matters even more stressful, it became impossible for me to continue driving back and forth to Rhode Island while attending to the hospital construction, preparing to open a brand new practice, and settling in to a new home. After three priceless years of mentoring by two dedicated practitioners whose example I hoped to live up to, I reluctantly said farewell to Dr. Jim Robbin and Dr. George Maurice. Both made it clear if I ever changed my mind they would welcome me back to the Warwick Animal Hospital. And with that, the family income dropped to zero.

By early June 1973, construction and equipping of the Shelburne Veterinary Hospital was 95 percent complete. I hired a wonderful young woman who had just graduated from the University of Vermont's four-year veterinary technician curriculum (no longer offered) to be my assistant. The rooftop heating/ventilating/air-conditioning unit was installed. I even included a personal touch to the sidewalk in front of the entrance door: Kin's and Penny's paw prints in the concrete.

I was eagerly anticipating opening the doors within the next two weeks when I received a call from Mrs. Joanne Myers, a Shelburne resident and cat owner. She had heard about the opening of my practice and wanted to know if I could help her sick kitty. The hospital was not yet quite ready for patients, but I was in no position to turn down my first client. I made a house call and examined Kitty Myers on the kitchen table.

I confess I do not remember exactly what Kitty's problem was, but I do recall we had a successful outcome and Mrs. Myers was pleased with the service. She promised to tell all her friends, and she paid me in cash. I took one of the dollar bills from her payment, framed it, and proudly hung it on the wall in my office. It was the beginning of thirty-seven years of continuous practice at the Shelburne Veterinary Hospital.

Steven B. Metz, d.v.m.

chapter seven

Building a Practice

Having survived my first appointment as the new doctor in town with Mrs. Myers and Kitty, I was ready to open the doors of my new hospital. I was proud of the Shelburne Veterinary Hospital in every way, except one nuisance problem. The roof leaked whenever there was a hard rain, which in turn damaged and stained the ceiling tiles. I called this to Frank Alling's attention several times, and his eventual diagnosis was that the leak was the fault of the heating/air-conditioning company. They needed to reset the entire rooftop unit—no problem, Frank assured me. He would contact the company and arrange for the required repair. Apparently, this was not a high priority on anyone's calendar, because several weeks went by with no action.

Meanwhile, clients were starting to trickle through the door. Some pet owners came simply to introduce themselves and see if this new doctor might be someone they could trust with the care of their beloved pet. Others came because of the convenient location or because their dog or cat needed "a quick shot, Doc." (I have always insisted that the term vaccination be used; shots are something you get in a bar. Anyone, I explained, could give a shot.) I gently explained that a physical examination was critical to the overall health of their pet. The real value of a veterinary visit is preventive medicine, teaching an owner to prevent illness, rather than coping with a disease or condition after it has developed. I spent considerable time with owners discussing nutrition, exercise, parasite control and prevention, and periodic blood tests to monitor kidney and liver function, among other health basics. Some owners were receptive to this approach; others were only interested in their pets' "shots." I did my best to answer the needs and wishes of an owner, but being young and earnest, I'm afraid I presented my ideas too strongly in some situations.

When an owner brought in a pet that was seriously overweight, I tried to emphasize how important it was to the pet's future health to correct the problem. Many owners just didn't take the problem seriously. They joked about how their pets loved their snacks and people food. Unfortunately, my response to this joking was to ask the amused owner, "Mrs. Jones, do you love your dog?" "Of course!" was the usual reply. "Then why are you killing him?" I demanded. As you might suspect, not all owners were prepared for this type of shock therapy; some didn't return to the Shelburne Veterinary Hospital. Word got out that Dr. Metz was good with animals, but rough on people. Fortunately, it didn't take me too long to realize that this was not a good way to get my point across.

I hadn't had my doors open for more than a few weeks when a large, young German shepherd was brought in by a Shelburne resident. The history given by the owner was that the dog had been lethargic for several weeks, and now he seemed to be having trouble breathing. No sooner did the owner get these words out of her mouth than the dog dropped to my reception room floor and started gasping. I called for my nurse and the two of us carried him back to the treatment area where I put an oxygen mask over his nose and prepared to start an intravenous drip. The dog stopped breathing. Listening for his heartbeat, I found none. I quickly gave him an intravenous injection of adrenaline (epinephrine) and began external heart massage, but it was no use. This dog had suffered a primary cardiac arrest. After several minutes of oxygen plus chest compression with absolutely no response, both the owner and I had to acknowledge the loss of this dog—my first loss after opening my practice a few short weeks before.

Not many diseases or conditions cause such a sudden death from acute cardiac arrest. Had such a thing happened at the Warwick Animal Hospital, the primary suspect would have been heartworm disease. Heartworm disease is a condition transmitted by mosquitoes, in which long worms migrate to the heart and some of the major blood vessels attached to the heart. These worms have the same effect as a large clot: They block the flow of blood to major organs, especially to the lungs. If diagnosed in time, it is treatable, although the medication used is quite toxic and must be used carefully. Heartworm was a relatively recent arrival in the Northeast at the time, and was believed to be spread only by salt-marsh mosquitoes; it was thought not to be a problem in northern New England, where the climate was colder. In Rhode Island, heartworm was quite common; I had successfully treated 126 cases during my three years at Warwick.

The most important thing about heartworm is that it is almost 100 percent preventable. A safe, inexpensive daily medication, diethylcarbamazine, was extremely effective in killing the young heartworm when a dog first became infected and before any damage was done to the heart or blood vessels. More recently, veterinarians have been prescribing a once-a-month medication, and there is even an injection that protects dogs for half a year.

When I first came to Vermont and met the area veterinarians, I asked whether heartworm was a problem. Without exception every practitioner told me that Vermont's climate was too chilly for heartworm; no salt marsh mosquitoes lived in our area. Not one veterinarian was testing dogs for heartworm. I did not believe there was no heartworm in Vermont for two reasons: Some cases had been found in Maine (plenty of salt marshes, but also a cooler climate) and in my senior year at Ontario Veterinary College, while assisting with the necropsy of two Ontario farm dogs who had never been out of the province of Ontario, we found heartworm (no salt marshes and a cool climate). If it could happen in Ontario, it could happen in Vermont.

The last thing I wanted as a new veterinary practice owner was a reputation as a troublemaker, so I hadn't questioned the beliefs of these practitioners when they insisted no heartworm was found in Vermont. I did decide to begin testing my canine patients for the condition with a simple blood test, but before I could begin testing, the unfortunate young dog from Shelburne expired in my reception area. From his heartbroken owner, I learned that this dog had been born in northern Vermont and had never been out of the state. Although the owner did not want a necropsy performed, I told her about my suspicion of heartworm and emphasized how important it was for the sake of the entire dog population in the state of Vermont. She reluctantly gave permission. I called the Department of Animal Pathology at the University of Vermont, where there were three veterinary pathologists. I explained the situation and asked for their help confirming my suspicion. Dr. Wes Bolton, senior pathologist at the laboratory, agreed to come to my hospital to perform the necropsy.

Sure enough, when we examined the heart of this unfortunate doggie we found several long white worms tangled in the valves of the heart. It was Dr. Bolton's first opportunity to see this condition; he was greatly surprised and thankful I had suspected heartworm. So far as we knew, this was the first case of heartworm in a native Vermont dog who had no chance in his short life to be exposed anywhere except northern Vermont. Dr. Bolton telephoned his laboratory and informed the other two pathologists of our findings. From then on, every dog necropsied at the University of Vermont Animal Pathology laboratory was carefully examined for heartworm.

I began contacting every veterinarian in the greater Burlington area to share my findings. Most practitioners were appreciative of my call, but a few were still skeptical, even though I made sure to say that Dr. Bolton, not I, had performed the examination.

Some area veterinarians acknowledged the finding but felt it was too rare to worry about—despite the fact that a dog had dropped dead in my reception room. It took several years for most practitioners to start testing for heartworm and prescribing the preventive medication.

The news was passed around the community in certain circles, among them the faculty of the University of Vermont College of Medicine. One afternoon I received a call from Dr. John Abajian, head of the Department of Anesthesiology. He was an avid duck hunter and the proud owner of Char, a middle-aged Labrador retriever, with whom he had enjoyed many successful hunts. Dr. Abajian had heard that heartworm was now a threat in our area and wanted to take absolutely no chances with his precious Char. He wanted to bring Char right down for a heartworm test. "Certainly, Doctor," I replied. "We'll do it right away."

I was thrilled to receive the call; Dr. John Abajian was the anesthesiologist who had pioneered the development of halothane—the most widely used inhalation anesthesia in human surgery at that time, and increasingly used in veterinary surgery. I had been using halothane as a surgical anesthetic since I graduated from school, and had purchased the same model of anesthesia machine Dr. Abajian used for his patients. Now this world-famous anesthesiologist trusted me with the care of his best hunting buddy. What an honor!

I was prepared to give him a grand tour of my new hospital, including my anesthesia set-up, but he appeared to be in a hurry and was not inclined to chat, even when I told him I used halothane and considered it a privilege to help him. I took a small blood sample from Char's front leg for the heartworm test and promised to call Dr. Abajian as soon as I had the results. He departed rather brusquely.

Forty-five minutes later, Dr. Abajian called back. "What did you do to my dog?" he growled. "He's having seizures. I'm bringing him right over."

Imagine how I felt: My first patient owned by a faculty member of the College of Medicine—and a famous one at that—was having some sort of problem immediately after I took a blood sample. Taking a simple blood sample could not cause seizures in an otherwise healthy dog, but the fact remained that Char had been perfectly healthy and happy before I laid hands on him, and soon afterward began having seizures. There goes my reputation in the community, I thought.

Shortly, Dr. Abajian drove into my parking area, and I met him at his car. I was quite nervous about my ability to solve Char's seizure problem, because the cause of seizures is often difficult to identify. In humans, sophisticated tests such as an electroencephalogram are often required. When Char jumped out of the car I noticed he was salivating profusely, the pupils of his eyes were constricted to pinpoint size, and instead of actual convulsions he was twitching—like an exaggerated shiver. When I put these three clinical signs together, I identified the probable cause: organophosphate poisoning. Organophosphates are a class of insecticides commonly used around outdoor gardens; poisoning of dogs and cats was not a rare occurrence.

I took Char's leash and brought him into the hospital. I was no longer concerned about making a good impression on Dr. Abajian; Char needed an immediate injection of atropine, which would block and reverse the effects of the poison in his system. Forgetting to whom I was speaking, I told Dr. Abajian, "Please hold him steady while I give him this injection," and I drew up the proper dosage of atropine.

"What are you giving him?" demanded Dr. Abajian.

"This is atropine; I believe your dog has organophosphate poisoning," I answered.

"Impossible!" he declared. "He's never out of my sight."

Again forgetting that I was contradicting a famous anesthesiologist, I said, "Well, I'm going to give it anyway." Dr. Abajian's jaw dropped. As I later found out, he was the absolute terror of the Departments of Anesthesiology and Surgery! When he issued an order, everyone ran—not walked—to carry it out.

I gave the atropine intravenously to Char. Within two minutes, his violent shivering and his drooling started to subside. To my great surprise, Dr. Abajian threw his arms around me and gave me a bear hug.

"I don't know how you figured that out," he said, "but you were right. Thank heaven, Char is going to be okay." We watched him for several more minutes, and gradually all his signs disappeared. While we were observing Char, Dr. Abajian remarked, "At some point, maybe I could help you set up a halothane anesthesia machine in your surgery room."

"Thank you, but you don't need to do that, sir. Let me show you what I'm using."

When he saw I was using the same machine he had developed and that he himself used, well, I definitely received the stamp of approval.

"Isn't there something I can help you with to show my appreciation?" he asked.

Half-jokingly, I said, "You know, if you happened to have a stray cardiac monitor lying around, I could certainly put it to good use." An instrument like that was definitely not in my budget.

Dr. Abajian left the hospital soon afterward, with Char trotting happily by his side; I promptly forgot about the cardiac monitor. Two hours later, Dr. Abajian called to let me know that the mystery of Char's organophosphate poisoning was solved. He had gotten into the neighbor's compost pile, to which some fertilizer mixed with insecticide had been added. I was relieved to hear that my diagnosis had been verified, and Dr. Abajian assured me that Char would have no further opportunities to get into such troubles. Two or three weeks later, a short, slight woman came into the hospital struggling with a large, heavy box. I came to the front desk and greeted her; she introduced herself as Mrs. Abajian, saying that John asked her to deliver the package. I said I couldn't imagine what it might be. She seemed quite surprised to hear it. "He promised you a cardiac monitor, didn't he?" she asked. "There it is."

I was flabbergasted! Such an instrument, even an older model such as this one, was expensive. "Please thank the doctor for me," I stammered. I had no idea he had taken me seriously. Mrs. Abajian shook her head. "I think he'd rather a member of his family take sick than for something to happen to that dog." It was the beginning of a close relationship to the Abajian family that has lasted all these years.

All did not go quite so smoothly at the new Shelburne Veterinary Hospital, however. One of the new clients was Roz Graham, editor of the local weekly newspaper. She was from Canada and familiar with the Ontario Veterinary College. She had a large, good-looking male Siamese cat who needed to take medication in pill form. Unfortunately, as good-natured as the big fellow was about everything else, he hated pills. But I was a relatively new graduate with all the latest techniques. "I can pill just about any cat," I assured Roz. She was clearly skeptical, but in her understated way, she invited me to demonstrate my method.

Cat lovers can anticipate what happened next. Any veterinary practitioner who works with dogs and cats would rather handle an angry 150-pound Saint Bernard than an uptight six-pound housecat. Dogs have one major weapon: their teeth. If the veterinarian can get a muzzle on the dog, no serious damage can occur. Take away a dog's ability to use his teeth and you can usually accomplish any treatment, with or without the administration of a sedative or anesthetic. Cats are an entirely different proposition. To begin with, they not only have an extremely sharp set of teeth but a set of dagger-like claws on each foot.

There are cat muzzles, but cats have relatively short noses, and the cat muzzle covers the eyes as well as the jaws. If the kitty is not already angry, putting one of these muzzles on will complete the job.

In addition to teeth and claws, the reaction time and speed of cats is almost unmatched throughout the animal kingdom. Once, an unsuspecting owner was stroking her apparently relaxed cat as he was sitting on the examination table. I had not even approached this cat. Suddenly, in a quick flash of cat fur, the owner jerked her hand away; the cat remained sitting on the table in the same position as before, still relaxed. But the owner and I were alarmed to see blood dripping from her arm; on examination, she had no fewer than four separate bites and two deep scratch wounds on her arm. The whole thing had taken less than five seconds, and neither of us had a chance to react before it was over. We were both stunned by the speed and ferocity of the attack. I wrapped the cat in a large bath towel and quickly put him back in his carrier, then dispatched one of my nursing staff to drive this owner to the hospital.

The final advantage a six-pound house cat has over us clumsy humans is flexibility. They are surely one of nature's most skilled contortionists; they can assume positions that would put a lifelong yoga practitioner to shame. Re-straining a cat for treatment of any kind is a true art form. I am convinced that some people are born with this ability, and others can work at it for years and still not achieve success. If you are skilled at working with cats, amazing things can be accomplished—one of my technicians developed the ability to take a blood sample from the jugular vein in the neck with absolutely no help and no restraint. The cat had to be a reasonably good-natured patient, of course, and some cats are simply unmanageable in a veterinary hospital setting. In these cases, the practitioner's only recourse is to administer an anesthetic to com-plete a treatment or test.

In the case of Roz Graham's cat, I was convinced I could easily give him his pill. I placed the palm of my left hand on the top of the cat's head, my thumb at one corner of the mouth and index finger at the other corner—thus forming an arch over the cat's nose. Next, I tilted the head back until the cat's nose was facing the ceiling. Taking the pill in my right hand, I pushed down on the center of the lower jaw to open his mouth. So far, so good, I thought, although I could feel the big fellow tensing up. The next step was to drop the pill way in the back of the throat in the center of the tongue and quickly close the cat's mouth with his head still pointing upward. All this had to be done with no hesitation.

At the exact moment I was to drop the pill into our feline friend's mouth, an explosion took place on the exam table. When the dust settled, the pill was on the floor, the cat was sitting in the middle of the table looking pleased with himself, and I was contemplating the lesson in humility I'd just been given. With the barest trace of a tolerant smile, Roz said, "No matter who attempts it, that has always been the outcome"—thereby absolving me from any sense of personal failure. This cat was a sweetie in every other way, but he was completely unpillable. A few years later, a gel was developed that could be mixed with certain medications to allow them to be absorbed through the skin. What a treasure for practitioners working with cats!

My next milestone was making the acquaintance of the Vermont Department of Fish and Wildlife and the area game warden. One morning a gentleman stopped in with a rather limp, sleek brown weasel-like creature he had hit with his car. Although I had never been up close and personal with this species, I immediately recognized it as a mink. It was unconscious but breathing well, with no obvious wounds. I felt all four legs and could discern no fractures. I carefully opened the mouth and observed the tongue was pink—a rough indication that no serious internal bleeding was occurring and that blood pressure was reasonable. My working diagnosis was concussion. I had never treated a mink before, but the principles of head trauma treatment are the same throughout the animal kingdom.

I tried but was unable to put an intravenous catheter in the tiny veins I could find. So I gave an intramuscular injection of dexamethasone, a potent corticosteroid, and placed hot water bottles next to the mink; his temperature was below what I expected of an animal with a relatively high rate of metabolism. To my great delight, within thirty minutes the little fellow began to show signs of recovering consciousness. I wrapped him in a heated towel and put him in a cat-sized compartment in my hospital ward. Now that I thought he had a reasonable chance to recover and be released, I called the nearest fish and wildlife warden, a Mr. Hislop, and told him I had a mink in my hospital with a concussion. He was showing signs of recovery, and I asked Mr. Hislop if he would help with the release when the mink was well enough to travel.

I was expecting some sort of encouragement or thanks for my efforts on behalf of this wild creature, but instead Mr. Hislop was angry with me.

"Do you have a license to handle wildlife?" he demanded. "You could be slapped with a big fine for your actions, you know."

I had used my staff, my hospital facilities, and my medication to help this animal, and the last thing I was about to consider when presented with an injured animal was proper licensing. It was not as if I were someone without proper medical training. Certainly, neither Warden Hislop nor anyone else in his department could have done any more for this mink. The more I thought about it, the angrier I got.

"If you think I've done something improper, then please come to my hospital and take this animal off my hands."

He assured me he would be right over. Within the hour, Warden Hislop came marching into my hospital. I made no attempt to introduce myself but led him straight to the mink's compartment. By now we had an entirely different animal. Mink are well known to be ferocious hunters and defenders of their territory. Although this fellow was still somewhat wobbly on his legs, he was acting more and more like a normal mink with each passing minute. I was interested to learn exactly how Warden Hislop was going to remove this lightning-fast streak of brown fury from the compartment. I stood well back and offered no help. As Mr. Hislop reached for the latch to open the cage, the mink bared its teeth and lunged at his hand. Fortunately for our game warden, Mr. Mink's aim was a little off due to his wobbly legs and head. Even so, he came within inches of having a piece of thumb-steak for breakfast. Warden Hislop hastily withdrew his hand and backed away from the cage.

"Maybe I'd better leave him here until he's feeling better. I'll come back for him in a few days." And with that, he left the hospital with no further discussion of any penalty or criticism leveled at me.

The next day, the mink seemed to be fully recovered, and was racing around the cage. I called Warden Hislop and left a message; I intended to insist he remove this wild creature from my hospital and release the mink back into the wild where he belonged. I waited all day for a return call, and when none came, I decided to take matters into my own hands. I carefully maneuvered the mink into a plastic cat carrier, put him in my car and drove out to Huntington, where he'd been hit. When I put the carrier on the ground in a patch of woods near the river and cautiously opened the door, a streak of brown fur emerged and the little fellow was gone. I wished him luck as I drove back to my hospital, and prepared for some more angry charges from the game warden. If he'd been upset with me for trying to save the life of this mink, I imagined my crime of setting the animal free without the warden's blessings would be considered even more terrible. I never did get a return phone call from the warden, nor did I hear any more about getting into legal difficulties because I did not have the required permit to handle and treat wildlife.

That was my introduction to the Vermont Department of Fish and Wildlife. Over the years, I have often worked with state and federal wardens and wildlife personnel, and the relationship has almost always been one of mutual respect and understanding. Rules and regulations governing who may handle and work with wildlife may seem overly burdensome or unnecessary; however, without these regulations, people who are neither qualified nor knowledgeable in helping wild species could do much damage and cause unnecessary suffering for wild creatures. Every spring we veterinarians get dozens of calls from well-meaning people who have found an "orphaned" baby bird on the ground or in the bushes. Because the adult birds are not with the baby, these folks conclude the young ones are orphans, not realizing that as long as they are standing right there, the parent birds will not come. So these well-meaning people remove the bird from its surroundings—and now they do have an orphan. Their next step in rescuing the baby bird is to try feeding it bread and milk. These two foods are apparently magical in the eyes of the public. The only problem is that birds do not drink milk, and bread has limited nutritional value, especially if the baby bird happens to be of a species whose normal diet is insects or berries. Then, everyone professes that once a person touches a wild bird, the human odor will prevent the parents from having anything more to do with the baby—wrong! Most birds have a poor sense of smell.

Little do rescuers realize that parents do not generally abandon a baby who has fallen out of the nest, or that in many cases spending a few days on the ground or in bushes is a normal part of maturation for the young bird. They are called branchers at this point in their development.

At this early stage of my growing practice, every day presented a new challenge. One of the most enjoyable aspects was meeting the fascinating pet owners: medical doctors, dentists, attorneys, teachers, nurses, IBM employees, farm owners, and many young families who often were as new to pet ownership as they were to parenthood. Not infrequently, I found myself in the role of family counselor.

I recall one visit by a young mother with her new puppy and her five-year-old son. Puppy was getting the first of the series of vaccinations that would protect against the most serious viral diseases to which dogs are susceptible. As I completed my physical examination and began to draw the vaccine into a syringe, the young fellow, who had been interested in the examination procedure up to that point, began to back away, saying repeatedly, "Not for me, not for me." His mother explained that the next day her son was to have a visit with his pediatrician to receive a vaccination. In an attempt to allay the boy's fear, I told him, "You watch your doggie and see if it hurts. I'm going to give him a painless vaccination and he won't mind one bit." I sprinkled a little puppy food on the examination table, and while the puppy was enjoying this treat, I gently inserted the needle underneath the skin and gave the vaccine in the space between the muscle layer and the skin. This is called the subcutaneous space, and is usually an area that is not particularly sensitive. Unfortunately, we humans do not have a significant subcutaneous space, so most of our vaccines are given in the muscle layers, which is definitely more uncomfortable.

It is, of course, still possible to minimize the discomfort of an injection by using the smallest size needle possible, using an area of the body that is least sensitive, and being gentle. Many of us have received an injection from a doctor or nurse who act as if they are throwing darts at a wooden board. A nurse told me that in school they practice on an orange.

When the five-year-old saw his puppy still wagging his tail and giving the doctor enthusiastic kisses, he ran over to the doggie and gave him a hug. I said to him, "Now when you go to your doctor tomorrow, you tell him you want a painless vaccination just like Dr. Metz gives." I never dreamed that he would quote me verbatim.

Two days later, the telephone rang and my nurse told me it was Dr. Jack Murray asking to speak to me. I didn't know a veterinarian by that name, but picked up the phone. "Hello. My name is Jack Murray and I'm a pediatrician in Burlington. What is this nonsense about painless vaccinations you've been feeding my patients? You're causing me a lot of trouble!" I was new in town, and the last thing I wanted to do was alienate a member of the medical community. As I started to stammer an apology, the other end of the line exploded in laughter. Dr. Murray, as it turned out, had a great sense of humor and had gotten quite a charge out of being held to the standards of a veterinarian. I was relieved I had done no damage to my professional reputation, but I certainly made it a point to be careful about what I recommended to another doctor's patient—human or non-human.

I confess that the behavior of some of the children who came to my hospital with their parents was foreign to the way my acquaintances and I were brought up. One young mother brought her two daughters along for an appointment with the family cat. While she sat watching, her daughters (ages nine or ten) got busy drawing pictures on my examination room floor with their crayons. My nurse and I spent part of our Sundays each week scrubbing the floors, and I was astounded that this mother did absolutely nothing to correct her children. I stopped my examination of the cat, asked the children to please stop using the floor, gave them some paper for their picture drawing, then got a scrub brush and cleaned the floor—all while the mother sat calmly and watched. I could detect no trace of embarrassment at all.

Another young mother brought in a young dog in thin condition due to a poor diet, consisting mostly of table scraps. He harbored a heavy burden of intestinal parasites, some of which this poor doggie had spit up on her living room rug. That convinced her that her puppy needed help. But it was she who needed help to understand the nutritional requirements of her dog. Unfortunately, she also brought her six-year-old son with her. Every time I tried to speak to Mom about the major changes she would have to make in feeding and managing her dog, this obstreperous boy would shout at the top of his lungs. I simply could not communicate. The mother shrugged her shoulders helplessly and said, "I just don't know what to do with him when he gets this way. I'll have to come back another time." The puppy was very sick and needed help immediately, not some other time when a six-year-old boy decided to permit it. I walked over to the boy's mother so I could be heard over the shouting and asked, "Would you like me to help? I promise not to hurt him in any way."

She nodded. "Yes! Please!"

I walked over to the boy, put my face right up to his, and told him, "You have to stop shouting. You're scaring your puppy, and I need to talk to your mother about him. One more shout and I'll have to put you in one of my cages like a wild animal. How would you like that?"

Just as I thought he would, the defiant boy said, "I wouldn't mind being in a cage. It would be fun."

"Really? Let's go." I held out my hand. To the mother's complete amazement, the boy took my hand (and my dare) and walked back to the ward area of the hospital with me. I lifted him up, put him in a medium-sized compartment, slid the locking bar closed, and walked out of the room without a backward glance. When I first put him in the compartment, he was grinning and quite cheery. By the time I got back to the examination room, there was dead silence from the ward.

"Is he okay?" his mother asked anxiously. "You didn't scare him, did you?"

In the worst way, I wanted to tell her that her little angel needed a serious scaring. But before I could say anything, the boy called out, "Dr. Metz! Dr. Metz! Come let me out! Let me out!"

I walked back to the ward, and through the bars of the compartment, I said, "If I let you out, will you promise to sit in the chair in the examining room and not make one sound?"

"Yes," came the quick reply.

"You're absolutely sure?" I asked, looking directly at him and making sure he was looking directly back at me.

"I promise," he said.

I unlocked the compartment door, lifted him down, and walked him back to the exam room. I pointed to the chair, and without any argument, he climbed up and sat.

"Now," I said, "we can discuss what needs to be done to help your puppy." The mother's jaw was already dropping when I pointed to the chair and the boy sat down with not a word. During the ensuing fifteen-minute conference, she kept sneaking looks at her transformed son. The boy kept his promise and didn't make a sound the whole rest of the visit. As the family prepared to leave, the mother turned to me and said, "I have a younger son at home. Could I get you to make a house call to treat him, too?" I just laughed and said that I'd be happy to help, but had a full appointment schedule right at my office. In subsequent visits, the young mother came without her children, so I had no further chances to evaluate my amateur psychological treatment, but at least I was able to complete an important consultation.

I did not earn such high marks during the next challenge I faced. One morning a rather unkempt-looking man walked into my office with a beagle trailing behind on a length of clothesline. The little dog was walking on three legs, carrying one hind leg up off the ground. Before I could even greet the man, he said, "How much to fix this?" I was accustomed to discussing finances with pet owners, but not usually before saying hello. A bit flustered, I didn't even ask what had happened to cause the injury.

"It depends on what the problem is. The leg may be broken. I'd have to take an x-ray to find out if it's broken, and if so, exactly where, and how badly."

"An x-ray, eh? How much would that cost?" I told him it would be about $15 (this was in 1973). "Fifteen dollars! A bullet only costs a nickel," he sneered.

Suddenly, I started to see red. Here was this poor doggie with a leg so badly hurt that he couldn't even put it down, and this owner was comparing the cost of veterinary care with shooting his dog. I could have understood if he decided to have the dog put to sleep, but to flaunt the thriftiness of shooting the dog— well, I'm sorry to say I lost my temper.

"Why, you cold-blooded son-of-a-bitch! The bullet would be better aimed in your direction," I told him. Without another word, he turned and walked out, the little beagle trailing after him on his three good legs. I later found out he had taken the dog to a nearby river, tied a large stone to the clothesline and dropped the dog into the water. Because I never learned the man's name, there was no way I could charge him with animal cruelty. Almost forty years later, this episode still haunts me. I lost my temper, became self-righteous, and who suffered? Not the terrible owner, and not I, but the patient—the one about whom I had sworn a professional oath to "First, do no harm." I never forgot the lesson: My primary concern must be the welfare of the patient, not my professional ego or sense of outrage. I'm sure this clear realization of my obligation to my patient first, and then the owner or client contributed greatly to my reputation of being rough on pet owners. Tact and grace were not my strongest suits.

As my practice grew, it became more and more difficult to make house calls. It didn't make sense to leave a well-equipped hospital, with all the instruments and all the medications I might need, get into an automobile, drive for a half-hour, and then try examining and treating a sick patient. In the typical home I found nothing approaching a suitable examination table; kitchen counters and kitchen tables were the most common substitutes, and insufficient lighting was especially troublesome. When I received a phone call from Mrs. Joan Foster asking if I would make a house call for her Newfoundland dogs, initially I tried to talk her into bringing them to my hospital. Her reply was, "You don't quite understand. I have twelve of them."

Newfoundland dogs have very long black hair, are huge (120-140 pounds), often slobbery, and usually friendly. When a Newfie did come into my hospital, I could pretty much count on a full vacuum cleaner bag and a thorough washing of my face and the exam room walls afterward. I finally agreed to go to Halirock Kennels to vaccinate and heartworm-test all twelve of Mrs. Foster's Newfoundland show dogs. As I drove up to her home, which was only a few miles from mine in Shelburne, I had a picture in my mind of what a breeder of Newfoundland dogs must look like. She would be large and strong, a prerequisite for managing these energetic giants. I was more than a little surprised when a slim, elegant woman came to the door and invited me in.

Joan Crile Foster's father, Dr. George Crile Jr., was a staff surgeon at the Cleveland Clinic and internationally recognized for his medical writing. Her grandfather, Dr. George Crile Sr. was a founder of the Cleveland Clinic and an internationally recognized surgeon. On her mother's side, that family owned the largest, most elegant department store in Cleveland. Joan's husband, Dr. Roger Foster, was a noted surgeon in his own right and became Director of the Vermont Cancer Center. He started the organ transplant program at the Medical Center Hospital in Burlington specializing in kidney transplants. Despite this distinguished background, Joan and Roger Foster were as unpretentious as they could possibly be. Most of the time Joan wore a loose floppy flannel shirt and a pair of jeans—a sensible saliva-shedding style if one is around twelve Newfoundlands much of the day. One evening at a concert I saw Joan dressed up, and she was a stunningly attractive woman—so much so that at first I didn't recognize her.

Joan's energy level was such that she could go back and forth through a swinging door all in one swing. I had to run to keep up with her. But it was her professional ethics for which I so admired and respected her. No matter how many dollars she might be offered for a puppy, she positively would not sell one of her dogs to anyone she had not met, and of whom she did not completely approve. It was not unusual for one of her puppies to sell for over a thousand dollars.

I was in her kitchen on a day when she received a phone call from a young couple who had recently purchased one of her pups after waiting many months for a Halirock dog. Through no fault of theirs, the young dog got out of their house, was hit by a car, and was killed instantly. I saw Joan's eyes fill with tears. She told the woman on the phone, "Don't feel so awful; when you're ready, I have another puppy I will give you." And one month later, that's exactly what she did, even though the puppy she gave them was one she had planned to keep and show. No amount of storytelling about Joan Foster can adequately describe her sheer vitality, quick wit, and common-sense approach to life. Later in her life, when she twice had to face a diagnosis of cancer, she was an inspiration to her family and all her friends and acquaintances—including her veterinarian.

This was the woman who invited me into her kitchen to treat her internationally renowned dogs. As I have mentioned, the test for heartworm involves taking a blood test. The most commonly used vein is the cephalic vein, which runs up the front surface of the front leg. Unfortunately, Newfoundlands have an extremely thick coat. (Joan often collected the hair and made attractive hats and scarves from it.) Not only could I not see the vein, as I usually could in a short-coated dog, but I often had trouble even feeling the vein due to the hair and the large muscle mass of the leg. My task in drawing the blood sample would have been ever so much simpler had I clipped some of the hair away from the vein area, but these were show dogs. No clipping could be done except in an emergency.

"Come on, Dr. Metz," Joan would challenge me. "Surely you can hit these great big veins first try."

I should mention that a large nerve runs up the leg quite close to the vein, so if one misses the vein and hits the nerve, even the sweetest dog will often resent the blood-drawing effort. During my first visit to Halirock Kennels, I was able to draw blood samples from the first eleven of these good-natured giants with a minimum of difficulty. I even collected several wet Newfoundland kisses along the way. Then came Dixie. She was a landseer Newfoundland; instead of the usual all-black coat, she had some flashy white markings on her chest and shoulders. Joan had purchased Dixie from another Newfoundland breeder for the purpose of outcrossing, which means incorporating different bloodlines into a breeding program. It is usually done to prevent breeding animals too closely related, and adds desired characteristics to future offspring. I cannot comment on which characteristics of Dixie's Joan wanted to add, but after several minutes trying to calm her down so I could take the blood sample, I certainly could have suggested a few that I hoped Joan didn't want to add.

Dixie had springs in her legs and in her rear end. The closest I can come to describing her is as a giant black and white rubber ball. She positively bounced. Finally, although Dixie outweighed Joan by about twenty pounds, Joan talked her into sitting still for a moment. No sooner had I positioned the needle in her vein and started to draw the sample, than she gave a giant leap over my left shoulder (I was kneeling on the floor in front of her). I had a firm grip on her front leg, so I too went sailing over my left shoulder—but hung on long enough to get the blood sample. Even Joan Foster was impressed.

Surprisingly, this event was not the high point of my first visit with Joan Foster. I inquired whether she had her dogs x-rayed for hip dysplasia—a crippling, inherited malformation of the hip joints seen in almost every breed of medium to larger dogs. It was a particularly common problem in the Newfoundland breed; any serious breeder had to make every effort to breed only dogs whose hips had normal conformation. The only way to evaluate the shape of canine hip joints was by x-ray study. The problem was so pervasive throughout the world of purebred dogs that a group of specialist radiologists formed an organization known as the Orthopedic Foundation for Animals (OFA). Breeders could have the films of their dogs' hip joints sent to this foundation for evaluation by at least three separate independent radiologists who then issued a consensus report on the conformation of the hip joints of the dog. If the dog's hip joints were judged to be of good conformation, the OFA would issue a certificate so stating, and the breeder could then advertise the parents of a litter of pups as OFA certified. This did not guarantee that the pups would absolutely have normal hips, but greatly increased those chances. If the grandparents of a litter also were OFA certified, chances of the puppies having normal hips were even better.

When I asked Joan Foster whether she had her breeding stock's hips x-rayed, she didn't answer, but led me to her bathroom. This was my first visit, and I certainly didn't know Joan well; I was a bit nervous when I followed her into the bathroom. I'm sure my jaw must have dropped in amazement when I entered the bathroom—because the entire room was wallpapered with OFA certificates. Joan burst out laughing.

In my forty years of practice, I have met many conscientious, even fanatical dog breeders, but never before or since have I seen or heard of anything like Joan Foster's bathroom.

Client by client, my practice continued to grow. I felt I had begun to develop relationships with the medical community, the University of Vermont Department of Animal Pathology, a major member of the dog breeder group in the area, and the Vermont Department of Fish and Wildlife (though I hoped to improve on my initial contact with the latter). My next opportunity to enlarge community relations came with a visit to my office by Dr. Janet Thomason— a soft-spoken local dentist. She brought her feline companion, an agreeable grey tiger cat, for annual vaccinations. Once more, the absolute necessity of a thorough physical examination was demonstrated during this visit. Here was a knowledgeable, educated owner, yet when I opened the cat's mouth as a standard part of my examination, I saw a large growth attached to the gum line next to the edge of the tongue. When I showed this to Dr. Thomason, she was mortified. She could not imagine why she had not discovered the growth herself. She felt quite ashamed and apologized to me for being a neglectful owner. I tried to alleviate some of her guilt by asking, "Are you in the habit of regularly examining your friend's mouth?"

"Unfortunately not," she answered.

"You have a lot of company," I told her. "Few cat owners open their cat's mouth and have a good look. And few cats are enthusiastic, or even cooperative about such an examination. I hope this is part of the reason you brought your friend to see me."

A few days later I surgically removed the growth, which turned out to be benign. The cat made a full recovery with no further mouth problems. To this day, whenever I see Dr. Thomason, she and I exchange greetings and recall the shock she received during her first visit to the Shelburne Veterinary Hospital.

As a bonus during this early period of my practice, I received a memorable reinforcement to the earlier lesson I learned about not assuming things. A sweet, elderly lady brought her adult female kitty in to see me because she noticed some flat white worms around her cat's rear, and she was quite alarmed. I reassured her that these worms—actually pieces of a larger tapeworm in her kitty's intestine—were not dangerous, just unsightly. Her cat had picked up the worm from eating either mice or fleas; these worms are not directly transmissible to people. Though tapeworm used to be difficult to get rid of, we now had a new medication effective in destroying them without making the cat ill. One minor problem was that this new medication only came in pill form, and the tablets were wrapped in foil to protect them.

I checked with the owner to make sure she could give her cat a pill, and she assured me she had given pills to her cat before. Her kitty was relatively accepting of medication in that form. With that assurance, I dispensed the medication with the following directions on the label: "Give one of the foil-wrapped tablets before the next meal today and one again tomorrow."

A few days later, the woman came into the Shelburne Veterinary Hospital and asked to speak to me. She had a question about the deworming medication. When I came to the front desk, she said, "Dr. Metz, I don't mean to question your prescription, but can you please tell me how it works? I gave the foil-wrapped tablets as per your instructions, but I noticed in the litter box that these tablets came out still wrapped in their foil. However do they work?" From that time on, whenever I dispensed medication of any kind, I showed the label to the owner, read the directions aloud, and went over the method of giving the medication to the pet. In many cases I actually demonstrated how to administer the medication, and asked if the owner had any questions about it.

Ever afterward, when I worked with a new veterinarian or nurse/technician I made sure to tell the enema story and the foil-wrapped tablet story so my elaborate precautions would not seem ridiculous.

As far as ridiculous scenarios go, I began to recognize one forming at my hospital facility. I had now been in practice several months, and my roof was continuing to leak. The heating/air-conditioning company had checked the situation and declared the problem to be the fault of the roofing company. After a delay of several more weeks, the roofing company inspected the area around the heating and air-conditioning unit and told me the problem was due to the structure supporting the roof, not the roof itself. When I relayed that opinion to Frank Alling, he laughed and told me the heating/air-conditioning company was just trying to avoid the cost and trouble of the repair; there was nothing at all wrong with the structure supporting the roof. He promised to speak with the roofing company and the heating company and resolve the issue.

Weeks went by with no action. As luck would have it, the weather was particularly rainy, and my ceiling tiles became more and more damaged. I was upset with all concerned: Frank Alling, the roofing company, and the heating/air-conditioning company. I had several conversations with each party, and no one seemed willing to assume responsibility and fix the problem. Finally, I'd had enough. I called Frank and the other two companies and arranged to have them all meet me at the hospital at the same time. I did not tell them that any-one else was coming. When they all had arrived, I set up a ladder and invited them to climb up on the roof with me to look at the situation. We all climbed up to the roof, and I kicked the ladder away so it fell on the ground below.

"Gentlemen," I said, "for months I've been getting the runaround from all of you. I don't know exactly what the problem is or who is responsible. I do know that the ceiling in my new building is getting ruined by continued leaking. Be-fore anyone leaves this roof, we are going to come up with a written and signed plan to correct this problem once and for all. I'm sorry if you're angry with me, but I've instructed my nurse not to pick up the ladder until this is done. So let's all cooperate and solve the problem."

At first, all three men thought it was a joke, but when I called down to my nurse and repeated my instructions, they began to take me seriously. As I suspected, it was more difficult for one person to blame another face to face. After only a few minutes, the accusations stopped, and a plan to repair my roof leak emerged, with all three gentlemen making suggestions and commit-ments to coordinate their efforts. Within one half-hour, the plan was finalized, written out, and signed by all three parties. I called down to my nurse, who set the ladder back against the roof edge, and we all climbed down. The roofer and the heating men told me I hadn't needed to resort to such tactics; they would have repaired the roof without being threatened, and they really didn't appre-ciate the way I had done business. Perhaps they were expecting an apology; instead, I reminded them of the months that had passed and all the shifting of blame. As for the man who was responsible in large part for the existence of the Shelburne Veterinary Hospital—despite his absence for much of the actual construction—Frank Alling waited until the other two men had driven away and then began to laugh so hard that tears were rolling down his face.

"Never in all my years as a contractor have I ever seen anything like that," he said when he could speak again. "Remind me to call you when I have another dispute between subcontractors."

Everyone kept their word and the roof leak and ceiling damage were finally repaired.

Steven B. Metz, d.v.m.

chapter eight

Adventures with my Vermont Colleagues

The practice of medicine, whether human or veterinary, is constantly changing. New medications are tested and become available. New diagnostic methods help practitioners find answers to perplexing health problems. Discoveries and techniques used in veterinary medicine are adapted, in some cases, for use in human medicine and vice-versa. These changes often occur so rapidly and frequently that one person has great difficulty keeping up, especially when that person is working fourteen to sixteen hours a day or more in a demanding medical and surgical practice.

One way continual education can occur is by collaboration with colleagues. I use the term colleagues, not competitors. At the Warwick Animal Hospital, I had four other veterinarians with whom to discuss cases, methods, and results. Here at Shelburne Veterinary Hospital, there were no such resources. When I introduced myself to the veterinary practitioners in the greater Burlington area, I hoped to foster the spirit of cooperation right from the outset. I approached the other veterinarians to see if we could work out coverage for after-hours emergencies. Until then, each practice had been responsible for emergencies occurring with their own patients. In multi-doctor hospitals this was not quite so tiring. In solo practices, even one after-hours emergency after a long day already spent at the hospital is exhausting, especially if the next day is fully scheduled.

After some discussion of the mechanics, Dr. Stokes' group (three doctors), Dr. Aliesky (a solo practitioner), and I set up a rotating emergency call schedule, which gave everyone more free time and much needed rest. As new practices opened in the area, they joined the coverage system. This cooperation paved the way for additional professional collaboration—to the benefit of pet owners and veterinary practitioners alike.

Shortly after I opened my practice, another veterinarian who had been in a mixed practice of both companion and farm animals for twelve years moved here from Pennsylvania. This veterinarian, Dr. Clinton Reichard, stopped in to see me; he told me he was opening a practice in Colchester, the town directly north of Burlington. He was temporarily using part of his house for his practice, but was planning to build a veterinary hospital on his property next to his home. We had much in common, and we quickly became the best of friends. We went to meetings together; we discussed cases on the telephone with each other; we argued about how to run a veterinary practice, and helped each other with difficult surgical cases.

In our first meeting, Doc Reichard asked me if I would let him use the plans I had drawn up for the construction of the Shelburne Veterinary Hospital as a guide for his new hospital. I was flattered that he liked my design, readily agreed to share my plans, and offered whatever else I could to help with his project. To my mind, this was just part of the nature of being a colleague. Dr. Reichard and I shared many adventures, which included his suffering through a rather brisk drive through the winding roads of northern New Hampshire in my little Volkswagen convertible on the way to a veterinary conference; the poor fellow had sufficient anxiety about my sporty driving that he wrenched the door handle right out of the door as he held on through a series of curves.

We both became members of two professional associations: the Vermont Veterinary Medical Association (VVMA), which comprised most of the veterinarians in the state, and the Tri-County Veterinary Society, which was more of a social gathering of veterinarians in the Burlington area. Through both of these organizations I came to know colleagues with whom I would otherwise have had little contact—particularly those from other parts of the state.

Many of these veterinarians had been in practice long before I entered veterinary medical college. At that time Vermont was primarily a rural state, and there was a preponderance of large (farm) animal or mixed (companion and farm animal) practitioners, as well as some veterinarians who specialized in equine practice.

At my first meeting of the Vermont Veterinary Medical Association I embarrassed myself over an issue about which I was far from the most knowledgeable or experienced practitioner in the room. Doc Reichard and I travelled to the Basin Harbor Club, a picturesque resort just south of the small city of Vergennes. He read an article to me from the latest Journal of the American Veterinary Medical Association. The article reported the terrible accidents involving racing thoroughbred horses and their jockeys resulting from administering phenylbutazone (commonly known as "bute") before a race. This drug is a potent anti-inflammatory painkiller; giving it to a horse before a race would mask the pain so that the horse would race as if there were no injury. This all-out effort on a leg or legs that were not sound sometimes resulted in horrible accidents when a horse stumbled or fell and the jockey was thrown. The sad results of these injuries was that the jockey was hurt, and all too often, the horse had to be destroyed.

Dr. Reichard had come from a mixed practice where he often worked with horses, so he was quite aggravated by this practice of giving bute to race horses. I rather casually said, "We ought to introduce a resolution at this meeting condemning this practice."

"Good idea," he said. "You and I will write the resolution and you read it at the meeting. I'll be right behind you." And before I could think about the possible consequences of such an action, that is exactly what happened.

I was a brand new member of the VVMA, three years out of school, not an equine practitioner, and I naively urged the entire Vermont veterinary community to declare public opposition to a practice in common usage by horse owners and their veterinarians. As I finished reading the resolution, dead silence filled the room for several moments. Then Dr. Clyde Johnson, an equine specialist with many years experience, said quite calmly, "Now Dr. Metz, we all understand how upsetting it can be to a young practitioner like yourself to read about these bad accidents. But as a professional organization, we wouldn't want to act too hastily on such an important matter."

I looked around the room for my friend and colleague who had been so excited about the matter in the first place—and who was going to be right behind me. I finally spotted him at the back of the room, next to the exit door, with his hand on the doorknob. After thinking it over, he had realized that more ground work needed to be done before such a resolution could be passed. I hardly blame him, but ribbed him unmercifully about his back-out tactics. By the time I turned back to the front of the room, Dr. Johnson had moved that our resolution be tabled pending further discussion. His motion was quickly seconded and passed with no dissenting votes I could see. I should have equipped myself with a lot more facts and figures, and perhaps consulted with some equine specialists before expecting the entire Vermont veterinary community to take the action I was proposing. Between unpillable cats and older and wiser colleagues, I was learning the value of experience, and yes, a little humility. More lessons followed.

During this same VVMA meeting, I made the acquaintance of Dr. Al Wright, who had been practicing mostly farm animal medicine in Vergennes for many years. He branched out into companion animal practice as the demand increased. Dr. Wright didn't seem to mind that I had opened a practice in Shelburne, but during lunch at the meeting, he did give a talk to us "young fellas," as he referred to any new practitioners. He reminded us that veterinary practice was not all there was to life, and that we would eventually have other community obligations to fulfill. He listed several community organizations of which he was a member, and stressed the importance of these types of obligations. Since Dr. Wright seemed to be more than a touch irascible when he referred to the "young fellas," I came away from the meeting hoping to stay on his good side.

Some months later, a farmer from the Vergennes area came to see me with one of his dogs. A few weeks earlier, this dog had cut his foot rather deeply on barbed wire. The owner had first taken his dog to Dr. Wright, who had examined and cleaned the wound, but he had not stitched or bandaged it, nor had he prescribed any antibiotics. The farmer soon noticed his dog was walking funny—as if he were on stilts. Also, his face had a funny look to it (the medical term is "rictus"), he ground his teeth when he tried to eat, and he could not open his mouth widely. This is commonly referred to as lockjaw. He was still able to drink water.

Recalling poor Henry, the Alaskan mule who died of tetanus, I noted that this dog's clinical signs were nearly the same. Fortunately, dogs seem to be far less sensitive to the tetanus toxin; actual cases of tetanus in dogs are rare with proper care of wounds. That is why dogs, unlike horses, are not vaccinated against tetanus. In my three years at the Warwick Animal Hospital, we had never seen a case. But here was a dog with a wound on his foot, living in a farm environment where tetanus bacteria are commonly found in the soil—contamination was inevitable. If the wound had been sutured and bandaged, and if the dog had been treated with antibiotics, tetanus almost certainly could have been prevented.

I told the owner what I suspected, but I was careful not to criticize Dr. Wright, emphasizing that tetanus seldom occurred in dogs. I hospitalized the poor fellow and started him on antibiotics, muscle relaxants, and tranquilizers, telling the owner that the next forty-eight hours would be critical. Fortunately, by the second day, the dog was able to open his mouth to eat, the muscle spasms in his face were relaxing, and his gait was more normal. I bandaged the wound and sent him home with continued antibiotics, cautioning the owner to keep him inside except when absolutely necessary. When the doggie did have to go out, the owner was to put a plastic baggie over the bandage to keep the

Steven B. Metz, d.v.m.

wound clean and dry. I emphasized no visits to the barn. After a few bandage changes and ten days on penicillin, the dog made a full recovery.

That was my first case of tetanus in a dog; I breathed a sigh of relief and hoped it would be my last. But only a few weeks later, in came a beautiful female pointer also owned by a farm family in Vergennes. This dog was having a great deal of difficulty walking and had not eaten in two days. It required little examination to see a large laceration running almost the entire length of her breastbone, about eight inches in length, with some areas showing exposed muscle tissue. The wound had occurred about seven or eight days earlier, and the dog had been examined by Dr. Wright, who had not sutured or bandaged the wound or prescribed antibiotics.

This dog's owner happened to have a good scientific background, as most successful farmers these days do. She asked me point-blank, "Could my dog have tetanus? And shouldn't this wound have been stitched?" Again, being careful not to criticize Dr. Wright's treatment of this wound, I replied that there was more than one way to manage wounds; however, due to the size and depth of this wound, I felt I should suture it, and place some drains so the wound could be irrigated with antibacterial solution. Meanwhile, since this dog wasn't able to open her mouth much, I would keep her from becoming dehydrated via intravenous fluids containing as many calories as I could safely include in the fluid solution. Once again, my treatment was large doses of penicillin (particularly effective against the tetanus bacterium), muscle relaxants, and tranquilizers. The wound was flushed twice daily. Again, after four days, this dog turned the corner, began to walk more normally, and was able to start eating soft food.

I removed the drains as the wound was starting to heal, instructed the owner to continue the antibiotics and keep the wound clean, and told her I would remove the sutures in ten days. Thankfully, this dog also made a full recovery. When Dr. Wright chanced to see the owner of this doggie on the street in Vergennes, he asked how the wound was coming along. She told Dr. Wright that her dog had gotten tetanus, that I had treated it, and that I had stitched the wound.

Dr. Wright scoffed, "I've treated hundreds of wounds without a problem. Dr. Metz didn't have to stitch that wound. It would have healed just fine on its own." When the owner brought her pointer back to me for suture removal, she told me that Dr. Wright had not hesitated to tell her that there was no need for me to have stitched this wound.

I had taken great care not to criticize Dr. Wright for his treatment of these wounds, which had resulted in a life-threatening infection in at least two cases. He was a far more experienced colleague who had made pretty clear his general opinion of young practitioners with limited experience, but the more I thought about his public belittling of my method of wound treatment, the angrier I got.

I have always believed that when two people have differences, they should talk those differences out. Particularly in the field of medicine, the wellbeing of the patient must take precedence over any one doctor's ego. Judging solely by the outcomes of his method of wound treatment, I felt Dr. Wright should at least be made aware of the consequences. I took a deep breath, picked up the telephone, and called Dr. Wright's office. He himself answered the phone. I identified myself, and then said, "You know, Doctor, I've treated two cases of tetanus in your patients who had wounds that you didn't suture and to whom you didn't prescribe antibiotics. I don't agree with those methods, but I was careful not to criticize you. I ask the same professional courtesy from you." Then I sat back, lifted the phone away from my ear, and waited for the angry response I expected.

Instead, to my complete surprise, Dr. Wright replied, "You know, young fella, I'm just as glad to have you up the road. I know that sometimes my methods are not the latest and I'm glad you called me." This was as gratifying to me as it was unexpected. Dr. Wright had treated me as a colleague and was a big enough person to acknowledge his error. I sincerely hoped that if I were ever in such a situation I would respond in exactly the same way—another important lesson to be filed away.

If throughout these stories I have in any way understated the importance of veterinary nurses, or technicians, as they are more properly titled today, I would be quite remiss. Veterinary technicians are vital to any successful veterinary practice; they are trained to do just about everything a veterinarian can do, except diagnose, prescribe, and operate. As I began practice, veterinarians were just starting to appreciate these talented helpers. Several schools throughout the country had a specific curriculum to educate veterinary technicians. The course of study was generally a two-year program, and a graduate received an Associate's Degree; graduates had little trouble finding a position at a veterinary practice.

Vermont had such a curriculum at the Vermont Technical College in Randolph. The college had chosen to title the course Veterinary Office Assistant. I had not had any contact with the school or its graduates because I seemed to have no problem having bright students from the greater Burlington area apply for any available position at the Shelburne Veterinary Hospital.

One day, two young ladies came to my hospital and introduced themselves as senior students at Vermont Technical College in the Veterinary Office Assistant program. They asked if they could observe my practice for the day, to which I readily agreed. I almost always enjoy working with students; besides, this would enable me to find out what these future veterinary technicians were being taught, and how they compared with pre-veterinary students at the University of Vermont, where many of my assistants were from. That morning I had a common surgical procedure to perform on a rather large young female German shepherd—an ovariohysterectomy. The anesthetic method I was using in the mid-1980s was to induce anesthesia with intravenous sodium pentothal, then place an endotracheal tube from the mouth into the first part of the windpipe, or "trachea." This is the same method used in human general anesthesia. The endotracheal tube ensures that the anesthetized patient has a constant supply of oxygen. Anesthesia is maintained with inhaled halothane through the same tube. Placement of this tube is a basic, essential skill that any veterinary technician should be able to perform; it was one of the first things I taught to all my assistants. So after I had anesthetized the German shepherd, I handed the endotracheal tube to one of the students and invited her to intubate the dog, who was sound asleep.

With a startled, almost horrified expression, she said, "Oh, no. I couldn't do that. We're not taught that type of thing." Nor had they been taught about monitoring general anesthesia during a surgical procedure. I was surprised. What kind of surgical assistance could these students give to a veterinary practitioner without such basic skills? As I questioned the students further about the content of their curriculum, I learned that the major educational emphasis was on filing, computer skills, and managing appointment schedules. I also learned that the students themselves were quite disappointed with the lack of technical veterinary content in their curriculum. Because of this disappointment, fewer and fewer students were choosing to register for this course of study. I didn't blame them for being disillusioned. I didn't spell it out for these students, but I felt their value to a prospective veterinary employer would be quite limited.

It so happened that my neighbor and good friend, Dr. Charles Bunting, was chancellor of all five Vermont state colleges. Only a few mornings after the visit from these students, he and I were taking a walk. He asked me if I was familiar with the Veterinary Office Assistant program at Vermont Technical College, and if so, what I thought of it. Poor Chuck Bunting! I'm afraid I turned the air quite blue as I told him how useless the curriculum was. He listened carefully, then told me only two or three students had signed up for next semester; he had to decide whether to abolish the course altogether, keep it as it was, or completely revise the curriculum. I told him there was a definite need for skilled veterinary technicians in Vermont and elsewhere, so I thought revision was the most sensible option. He then asked if I would be willing to help with the curriculum revision, and I agreed. Only two weeks later, I received a letter from the Office of the Chancellor appointing me as chairman of a committee to investigate the feasibility of completely revising the curriculum of the Veterinary Office Assistant program.

This committee consisted of Dr. Jon Stokes, a colleague in the Burlington area, and two members of the faculty at Vermont Technical College. There was also a third veterinarian on the committee, none other than my former polo coach at Cornell, Dr. Steve Roberts. Dr. Roberts' veterinary specialty was obstetrics and reproductive medicine. He had written the most widely used veterinary textbook on the subject in the United States, and he had the reputation of being a strict and demanding professor. He didn't bother to disguise his criticisms with flowery language, particularly when addressing the would-be polo try-out students. I remember one day at Cornell, he called me over after watching me ride in a scrimmage and said, "Metz, you're not a polo player, you're a g—d— cowboy. You're out!" Thus ended my brief career as a polo player. I admit that being dismissed in that manner smarted a bit, but in fact, Dr. Roberts was correct. I had spent a fair amount of time riding cow ponies, and even riding a bit in rodeos. Since then, Dr. Roberts had retired from teaching at Cornell and moved to Vermont to join his brother, who had a veterinary practice in Woodstock. As if that were not coincidence enough, Dr. Roberts had helped design the very curriculum our committee was about to dismember—and I, the young "cowboy," was chairman.

I introduced myself to Dr. Roberts, as I was sure he wouldn't remember our brief contact thirty years earlier, and we got right to work. We threw out almost the entire existing curriculum.

As the process of revising the curriculum proceeded, I became more and more uncomfortable with discarding Dr. Roberts' work of several years before. He himself seemed quite at home with the process and made many good and practical suggestions, but I still felt awkward in the role of chairman in the presence of such a distinguished member of my profession. Finally, after several sessions of our committee had passed, I went over to Dr. Roberts and said, "I don't suppose you remember me at all, Doc Roberts, but back about thirty years ago, you threw me off your polo team."

With a twinkle in his eyes, he replied, "I remember. I was just waiting for you to mention it." What a laugh we both had! And we continued working together for more than a year until the new Veterinary Technology curriculum was in place. The class swelled to twenty-five—maximum capacity—in one year. Today, it would be rare to find a veterinary practice in Vermont that does not employ a technician graduated from this program.

It was not only my veterinary colleagues with whom I collaborated. There were many times when human and veterinary medicine dovetailed, to the mutual benefit of both practitioners. In one experience, I ended up working with the departments of Rheumatology and Radiology at the Medical Center Hospital of Vermont. One day, I had a visit from an attractive couple who came for advice on what breed of dog they should have for their first pet. The gentleman was Dr. David Newcombe, a practicing rheumatologist, and his wife was Sissel, a tall, athletic Norwegian for whom the dog was to be a companion. They wanted an energetic easy to train dog that could go places with them.

Back when Connie and I were trying to choose a dog, my preference was the Doberman pinscher because of their trainability, their athleticism, and their usually stoic behavior when they needed medical attention. So I recommended they consider getting a Doberman. It turned out they fell in love with the breed and soon brought me a puppy that was a delight to play with and handle. Like any puppy, he was quite mischievous and inclined to chew various articles around the house. This puppy unfortunately took things a step further and ate a pair of Sissel Newcombe's stockings. Sissel was over six feet tall and so those stockings were not small. Nylon is totally indigestible, so the stockings formed a large intestinal blockage, and the poor puppy began to vomit anything he tried to eat.

Because puppies swallow things rather frequently, gastric or intestinal foreign material was high on my list of possible diagnoses, and I took a set of abdominal x-rays. Although soft and non-metallic objects do not show up clearly on plain x-ray views, the size and shape of the intestine is usually altered significantly and can be strongly suggestive of a blockage. Blockage treatment required some relatively major abdominal surgery, and because this was a young dog for which I felt somewhat responsible, I wanted to be as sure of the diagnosis as possible. I asked Dr. Newcombe if he happened to have a radiologist friend who would look at the films and give his opinion. This is how I met

Dr. Richard Heilman of the Department of Radiology at the Medical Center Hospital of Vermont in Burlington.

Dr. Heilman came to the Shelburne Veterinary Hospital and studied the abdominal films of the young Doberman. If the situation hadn't been so serious, I would have laughed out loud, because for the purposes of reading x-ray films, human anatomy is oriented top to bottom, whereas dogs are front to back. So the good Dr. Heilman spent the first few minutes holding the films first this way, and then that way, until the anatomy started to make sense. Eventually, he agreed that the films seemed to show an intestinal blockage due to a foreign body.

This was before the era of commonly available specialists. Our training in school, as well as my experience at Warwick, had theoretically equipped me for such a surgery, and the puppy clearly needed to have the stocking removed from his intestine. Dr. and Mrs. Newcombe agreed to the procedure, but, this being their first dog, their anxiety level was high—as was mine.

In some cases, removal of a foreign body from stomach or intestine can be fairly routine. In other cases, the foreign material can cause severe damage to a section of intestine. If that happens, the damaged part of the intestine must be removed and the healthy ends stitched back together in a leak-proof manner. This surgical procedure is called resection and anastomosis and is a completely different category of surgery.

Even if there is no serious damage to the stomach or intestine and the foreign material can be removed through a single incision into the affected area, the incision must be securely and carefully closed. This is not only to prevent leakage of intestinal contents into the abdominal cavity (which would cause severe inflammation and infection-termed peritonitis), but also to avoid narrowing of the intestine, thus creating a permanent partial blockage—from the very surgery done to correct a blockage.

All seemed to go well during the surgery, and I thought the intestine looked healthy, so I did not have to do a resection. Given the size of the stockings, I had to make a fairly long intestinal incision that required a lot of careful suturing for safe closure. Once the stockings were removed, both the Newcombes and I were quite ready to have the puppy jump up, start running around, and eating normally.

Unfortunately, recovery from such major surgery often does not proceed quite so smoothly. Various body tissues have been traumatized no matter how careful the surgeon may be, and the puppy had not been able to eat for two days prior to the surgery. When he didn't want to eat after twenty-four hours post surgery and was running a low-grade fever, I began to ask myself, Has the incision developed a leak? Could there still be some foreign material elsewhere in the gastrointestinal tract? Could there be a section of intestine that was not as healthy as I thought?

I took another set of abdominal films, and again called Dr. Heilman for his opinion. It must have been difficult for Dr. Heilman to decide who needed the most reassuring—Dr. and Mrs. Newcombe or me. He did his best, giving his opinion that there was no evidence of peritonitis at this early post-operative time. Radiologists look at shadows on a film: black shadows, grey shadows, and white shadows. If one grey shadow is greyer than another grey shadow, it could mean the difference between life and death. Often, the interpretation of an x-ray is quite subjective, and two radiologists can have entirely different opinions on what that film shows (or does not show). X-ray techniques themselves are not always reliable in revealing a disease process. That is why CT scans (CAT scans) and MRI techniques were developed and are in such wide use in human medicine today. Despite the great expense of the instrumentation, these techniques are being used in veterinary medicine at some universities and large veterinary centers more and more frequently.

None of these more advanced techniques were available back in the 1970s. So we all just had to wait to see how the puppy responded to supportive care: intravenous fluids, antibiotics, and pain medication. I brought a cot to the hospital and for two nights slept right beside the little fellow's compartment. On the third post-operative day, we all cheered when his fever broke, he stood up, and started to take an interest in food. I had to gently restrain Sissel Newcombe from bringing in sirloin steak for the young Doberman, although I was sure that when he went home on the fourth day, he found some extravagant fare in his doggie dish. I was also pretty sure that the Newcombe home was going to experience some major renovations to puppy-proof the living space.

A word to all new puppy owners: Just as with human babies, every new object that can fit in the mouth will go in the mouth, and it will often be swallowed. Over the course of more than forty years in veterinary practice, I have removed from dogs' stomachs and intestines such exotic objects as golf balls, fireplace gloves, pieces of rubber toys, the little bell or squeaker from some toys, coins, all manner of clothing—even a small butcher's knife. I have treated severe electrical burns of the mouth and tongue of puppies (and kittens) who have chewed electrical cords. I have had to wash out dogs' stomachs after they have swallowed their owners' medications. Some of these episodes have been in adult dogs, as well, but puppies are by far the most common victims. Cats seem to be more discriminating about what goes in their mouths. But they do have a great weakness for string, thread (with or without a needle attached), and yarn, all of which, if swallowed, pose extreme danger to the intestines. When cats do swallow these materials, it is a true emergency, and almost always requires major surgery.

I advise all owners of puppies and kittens to puppy- and kitten-proof their homes painstakingly. Walk around every room to which your puppy or kitten will have access, and remove anything the youngster can reach. Unplug lamp cords when you will not be home to supervise. Empty or remove trashcans; for some reason paper fascinates puppies and kittens. And when you are finished, invite a friend to look over the same rooms. After the Newcombe puppy's experience, I became an especially passionate advocate of pet-proofing one's home. A much easier way of preventing our companions from getting into such difficulties is a dog or kitten crate. I have heard people claim it is cruel to put a pet in a crate, though some of these portable compartments are quite luxurious. I agree that keeping a puppy in a crate for more than a few hours is inappropriate and results in poor socialization, poor mental development, and often causes difficulty in house-training. But the proper use of a crate can be a lifesaver.

My next exciting collaboration with a member of the medical community shifted to the field of dermatology. Through my door one afternoon came an elderly Mrs. Mary James, leading her black cocker spaniel, Jingo. His ears were bare and scabbed. The poor doggie was so itchy that he couldn't even walk from the front door to my examination room without sitting and scratching at his ears and chest, which was also losing hair. His owner was clearly upset about the condition of her dog's skin. As she began to tell me about her dog's problem, she stopped for a moment and said, "You know, Dr. Metz, I recently lost my husband to cancer. This dog is my only family now and we are quite close. He shares the couch with me, and even sleeps at the foot of my bed. Is it possible he has my condition?"

Then she told me that lately, she had been extremely itchy. She had been seen by one of our local dermatologists, who told her that her problem was nerves, the stress of losing her husband, and the stress of her job as a supervisor in a large grocery store in the Burlington area. This dermatologist had advised her to quit her job to reduce stress in her life. This advice was particularly difficult for Mrs. James to accept because she had only one more year to work to qualify for her retirement pension. By quitting now, she would lose the pension she was counting on for her retirement years.

At first, I was dumfounded by the dermatologist's diagnosis of nerves. After thinking about the situation for a few minutes, I realized I had a big advantage over that dermatologist; I was seeing the whole family. My role was more like the old-fashioned family doctor, in contrast to the specialist. It was the responsibility of that specialist to get a complete history, which certainly should have included any pets in the household. But it did not require a specialist to diagnose Jingo's problem. Few skin diseases cause such intense itching, and the bare and scabbed areas of the body completed the typical picture of sarcoptic mange, commonly called "scabies." This disease is caused by a tiny mite that irritates the skin and causes such intense itching that the poor patient is constantly scratching, thus causing hair loss and scabbing. This type of mange is contagious to humans, though many times the condition clears up spontaneously without treatment.

I asked Mrs. James if she had any rashes or spots on her skin. She rolled up the shirt cuff of her blouse and there at the wrist, I saw the telltale red spots typical of scabies in people. Another common area affected by the sarcoptic mite is the waist or beltline; during a visit with one itchy young woman and her itchy dog, I had to stop her from disrobing in the exam room to show me her spots. The condition usually responds quite well to treatment—the itching and scabbing resolves and hair grows back. The problem arises if the owner does not get treatment until the whole dog is affected. Then we must also treat the inevitable secondary bacterial infection and the course of the disease is greatly prolonged.

I started Jingo on treatment, which involved frequent baths with an insecticidal shampoo. I suggested to Mrs. James that she not quit her job just yet, and that she make another appointment with her dermatologist to confirm his diagnosis of nerves. I was extremely careful not to criticize the dermatologist or his diagnosis, but I did tell her that Jingo did not catch his skin problem from her; once his treatment was started, she could feel perfectly free to let Jingo on the couch or bed. As soon as Mrs. James left my office, I called the dermatologist and diplomatically let him know that I had just diagnosed scabies in his patient's dog. I concluded the conversation by saying, "I hope this information might be of some use to you." He thanked me for the call, and three weeks later, I received nice thank-you cards from both the dermatologist and Mrs. James, who reported that both she and Jingo were doing much better and that she didn't have to quit her job after all.

Scabies is just one of several conditions that, under the right circumstances, can affect pet owners. Some others are ringworm, intestinal parasites (especially in children), infections from bites or scratches, bites from fleas, Lyme disease from ticks carried into a home by dogs or cats, and rabies from the bite of an infected animal. Because people live so closely with their pets—Mrs. James' devotion to her remaining family member is a common example—professional communication between the family physician and the family veterinarian is often critical. It is a regular part of the curriculum for veterinary students to learn those diseases that are communicable from animals to humans—such diseases are termed "zoonoses"—and be familiar with the effects those diseases have on people.

Many, if not most medical schools, including the University of Vermont College of Medicine, have veterinarians on their teaching and research staffs because it often requires the combined knowledge and skill of both professions for the successful treatment of some illnesses. The case of Mrs. James and Jingo is only one example.

On a quiet morning at the Shelburne Veterinary Hospital, the door swung open without any warning and a young woman rushed in carrying her adolescent basset hound, Rudy. This doggie seemed to have his mouth open quite widely, but nothing was in his mouth to account for that position. The owner, who was almost hysterical, explained that this happened whenever Rudy yawned. Usually the jaw became unstuck after a few minutes, but not this time. I carefully felt the jaw joint and tried to gently manipulate it back to a closed position. Although Rudy didn't seem to be in pain, the jaw was absolutely immovable. There was only one thing to do, and that was to anesthetize Rudy so his muscles were relaxed; the anesthesia would allow me to use more force in unsticking the jaw joint without causing discomfort or pain.

Under a light plane of anesthesia, I was able to return the jaw to the normal, closed position. While Rudy was waking up, I asked the owner how often this happened; I was concerned to learn that the jaw often got stuck two or three times a day. Obviously, this owner couldn't rush her dog to the veterinary hospital for anesthesia every time Rudy yawned. Something was structurally wrong with one or both sides of his jaw joints.

The jaw joint, called the temporomandibular joint or TMJ, is not as complicated as some other joints in the body, but it is located in a tricky area, right near the middle and inner ear structures, one of the large salivary glands, and the large facial nerve that supplies the muscles of the face. You do not just casu-

S t e v e n B. M e t z , d . v . m .

ally operate on jaw joints without a great deal of expertise and experience. As it happened, the Burlington area was blessed with extraordinary medical and dental talent. Recently one of Burlington's oral surgeons, Dr. Paul Danielson, had collaborated with another veterinarian in the area and had made a new jaw out of a piece of rib for a red fox that had been hit by a car.

I called Dr. Danielson at his office and explained Rudy's problem. I told him I realized it was an imposition to ask that he remodel Rudy's jaw joint, but I also told him how upset the owner was and what a recurring problem this dog was having. Without hesitation, bless him, he agreed to do the surgery that night, as long as I could do the anesthesia.

That evening, I was truly fortunate to watch a surgical artist at work. After I anesthetized Rudy, Dr. Danielson was able to identify which joint was causing the problem by opening and closing Rudy's mouth and feeling which side was not properly aligned. He positioned the jaw so it became stuck open, and using my veterinary anatomy textbook, showed me the piece of bone in the joint that was improperly shaped. He surgically opened the joint, skillfully avoiding the large facial nerve and the salivary gland. With a pair of bone-cutting forceps, he quickly remodeled the bony component causing the problem. I didn't time the surgery, but Dr. Danielson was so quick and sure it seemed to take only a few minutes. Before putting in the closing sutures, he opened and closed Rudy's jaw several times. He put pressure on the joint from different angles and showed me that there was now no possibility of the joint becoming caught in the open position. One of the most inspiring aspects of working with Dr. Danielson was his complete enthusiasm for correcting a serious problem and making the jaw work properly. He didn't care one bit that his patient was a dog. In fact, I think he got pleasure out of working with a different type of patient and still achieving perfect results. A surgery of that type in humans would cost thousands of dollars; Dr. Danielson refused to take one cent for his service.

Only a few short years after I began practice in Shelburne, I had the chance to attend a joint conference between veterinarians and physicians in which problems common to both professions were discussed. The occasion arose because several times I was asked to examine cats that had bitten family members or visitors to a home; the cat bites were becoming badly infected a few days afterward, even though the bite victims had seen their physicians. Several times it was children who had been bitten, due to excessively rough handling of the family cat.

Just after this conference, I was taking our dogs out for their morning walk along our road. Our closest neighbor, Dr. Marshall Land, was a well-known pediatrician in Burlington, and when, this particular day, he stopped to say good morning, I mentioned to him that I had recently seen some cases of cat bites in children that had become badly infected, even though the children had been seen by their pediatrician. It was of particular concern to me, because infections from cat bites are almost always preventable with prompt treatment. Within a few days Dr. Land invited me to give "grand rounds" in front of the area's pediatricians on the subject of animal bites in general and cat bites in particular. Grand rounds was a regularly scheduled meeting at which some topic of medical interest or concern was discussed after a presentation by a guest speaker.

I don't know if this group of pediatricians had ever had a veterinarian speak, but I was determined to do everything I could to represent my profession in a way these physicians would respect and remember. I brought to the lecture hall, which was in the Medical Center hospital, my 90-pound Doberman. (After years of controversy, and after the loss of Kin, I finally did add a beautiful black-and-rust male Doberman, Tristan, to our household— over the strenuous objections of Connie.) I also brought Penny, our little six-and-a-half pound Burmese cat. I believe that was the first time a non-service dog or cat was permitted in the medical center.

As each pediatrician entered the lecture hall, I greeted them by showing them the size and shape of the teeth of each of my companions. Most of the group was quite nervous about getting so personal with the formidable dentition of Tristan, though he was as gentle as any pet I've ever owned or worked with. The doctors were not nearly as concerned about Penny's sharp little teeth, which was precisely the problem.

The fangs, or canine teeth, of cats are relatively small when compared to those of almost any dog. They are sharply pointed and cone-shaped. Because of the size and shape of these teeth, the bite wounds inflicted by cats appear as small puncture wounds that look harmless at first. That is the reason these wounds are not always taken as a significant threat by physicians. The rest of the story, though, is that cats carry in their mouths a certain bacterium, Pasteurella multocida, which is not harmful in that location but usually causes infection and abscessation if injected under the skin. This is especially likely if the wound closes to prevent air from getting to these bacteria. This is exactly what happens with a cat bite. The sharp teeth function just like a hypodermic needle to inject Pasteurella under the skin; the wound closes up quickly because of the shape of the teeth. Closure provides exactly the environment needed to form an abscess

S t e v e n   B .   M e t z ,   D . V . M .

and spread infection to the surrounding areas. Once that happens, treatment often involves surgical opening and cleaning out the wound area. By contrast, if the bitten person is given appropriate antibiotics within the first twelve to twenty-four hours, the surgery and drainage can almost always be avoided.

That was the message I hoped to convey to the pediatricians. After reviewing the information and realizing that I was not licensed or trained to practice human medicine, I took a deep breath and said, "Ladies and gentlemen, in my opinion every patient who has been bitten by a cat should immediately be put on a course of antibiotics." Then I stepped back from the microphone and watched the reaction of the audience. I saw one doctor turn to the one sitting next to him, saying, "I always do give antibiotics, don't you?" "No, I don't," replied the other pediatrician, "only when there actually is an infection present."

Within moments, the room started to buzz with small groups discussing what I'd recommended. Many doctors were concerned about the overuse of antibiotics, which was the reason resistant strains of bacteria were developing in many of the bacterial conditions physicians (and veterinarians) must treat. Some pediatricians felt local treatment of bite wounds, rather than systemic antibiotics, was all that was required. In some cases, the discussion was quite vehement and there were sharp disagreements. Several doctors came to the podium to voice their opinions. I never did get to finish my presentation, because of the heated discussion my recommendation had provoked. Afterward, Dr. Land told me that he couldn't remember a more intense discussion during grand rounds.

Several years later, I was asked to repeat my presentation to the pediatricians. I had the thrill of seeing our youngest son Jamie, who had just graduated from the University of Vermont College of Medicine (and who intended to make pediatrics his area of specialization), sitting in the lecture hall listening to his father give a scientific presentation to his professional group. It was an honor to be asked to speak in front of this group of dedicated physicians—and to be treated as their colleague.

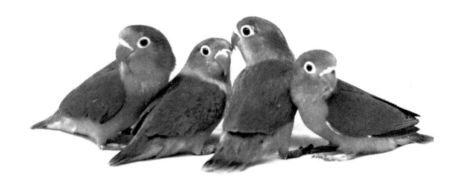

Matthew, Mark, Luke, and John are lovebirds, a particularly social and affectionate species of small parrot.

chapter nine

For the Birds

If I thought collaborating with my human medical counterparts was adventurous, my decision to include avian, reptilian, and small mammalian patients in my practice was a truly exciting challenge. My determination to care for wild birds, companion birds, snakes, turtles, lizards, chinchillas, guinea pigs, hamsters, rats, mice, gerbils, hedgehogs, and sugar gliders was also a rare opportunity to be a pioneer in our area. None of the veterinary practitioners in the entire northwestern part of Vermont, nor the adjoining area of New York State, was working with these species.

I am often asked, sometimes by veterinary practitioners themselves, why someone would bring their $15-20 budgerigar (often incorrectly called a parakeet) to a veterinarian for examination and treatment when it might result in significantly greater cost than the original price of the pet. Not to mention, if the owner of one of these lively and colorful creatures did bring a sick "budgie" to a veterinarian, what could that practitioner do to help? Everyone assumes that birds—especially small birds—are too delicate and not much can be done for them in the way of diagnostic testing or treatment.

I believe the answer to the first question not only pertains to birds, but also to every living creature, domestic or wild, with which humans have decided to concern themselves. The lowliest mouse, garter snake, and $15 canary or budgie has a value to the owner or caretaker far exceeding a purchase price. I cannot begin to tell how many clients have come to me with their tiny avian companions and made it clear that these creatures are family—sometimes the only family a person might have. Let me repeat the valuable lesson I learned during my time at the Warwick Animal Hospital: Never prejudge what decision a pet owner will make regarding the care of a patient. I will shortly give a convincing illustration of this principle.

Secondly, if we think about wild birds in their native habitat, we must realize that far from being delicate, they are tough creatures that survive storms, forage for food that is sometimes scarce, evade predators, and raise families. The persistent wives' tale that we must not allow a draft of air to blow upon a bird is, of course, the height of fantasy. Who protects birds from drafts when they are out flying around in the wild? I once watched a pair of Amazon parrots, whose native habitat is tropical jungle, have a grand time playing for a short while in the snow! I am constantly reminding overly protective bird owners that their feathered friends have a built-in down parka. It is clearly not correct to conclude that birds are overly delicate.

Likewise, it is foolish to assume that nothing significant can be done to diagnose and treat their illnesses. It is true however, that as a survival tactic birds hide symptoms of illness until they are too sick to do so. Thus, it requires an observant, knowledgeable owner to realize just when an avian companion requires medical attention. These days, with proper training, veterinarians can take x-rays of birds, do blood tests, endoscopies, and even perform sophisticated surgeries—all due to the efforts of dedicated researchers and practitioners.

In the 1970s and 80s, avian medicine was in its infancy. There were a few pioneers leading the way, treating avian illnesses, doing groundbreaking surgery, and investigating the effects on their avian patients of various medications used in dog, cat, and human medicine. One of these pioneers was Dr. Ted Lafeber, who had one of the first avian practices in the United States. In addition to being a practitioner, he was also an enthusiastic and inspiring lecturer on the subject of avian medicine. Because there were no readily available textbooks on the subject at that time, those veterinarians who were interested in avian medicine flocked to hear Dr. Lafeber speak.

I will never forget the first of many lectures by Dr. Lafeber that I was fortunate enough to attend. The meeting was held in one of the classrooms at the veterinary college at Cornell University. On each desk was a paper bag, from which a variety of bird sounds emanated. The more adventurous members of the audience opened the bags and discovered little Budgerigars, which promptly flew out of the bags and around the room before being gently recaptured.

Dr. Ted Lafeber stood at the head of the classroom with a wonderful wide grin and watched the audience discover his opening demonstration. When things settled down he asked, "Why would anyone want to keep a bird as a companion?" We waited. For the next thirty minutes, he listed and discussed the virtues of birds as companion animals, including their appealing colors, lively personalities, cheery sounds, hardy constitutions (with proper care), and their lack of requirement for outside exercise. He spoke, too, about what was known in the burgeoning field of avian medicine, surgery, nutrition, and general husbandry, as well as what, so far, was still unknown. The latter was quite a long list, and Dr. Lafeber insisted that it was our responsibility to keep up to date with new findings, which seemed to expand daily.

After attending one of Dr. Lafeber's daylong sessions, one could not help but be inspired to do everything possible for these intelligent, beautiful, exotic creatures. Listening to lectures, however, is no substitute for actual hands-on practice, and because most bird owners were not used to bringing their companions to a veterinarian, I was certainly not seeing many patients. I anticipated it would take several years and much public education to convince bird owners that a knowledgeable veterinarian could help their sick or injured pets.

Because of the relatively infrequent opportunity thus far to work with birds and the scarcity of published material on avian medicine, I was understandably concerned about how to gain experience and expertise. Luckily, one of the leaders in avian practice at that time—Dr. Margaret Petrak, affectionately called "Midge"—was on staff at the Angell Animal Medical Center in Boston, Massachusetts. Dr. Petrak was a pioneer in avian practice, and in 1969, she published the very first text on avian medicine in the United States: Diseases of Cage and Aviary Birds. Because Angell Animal Medical Center was the largest veterinary hospital in the Northeast other than New York's Animal Medical Center, Dr. Petrak's avian practice was likewise the largest avian practice.

Boston was a five-to-six hour drive from Burlington in good weather, but the travel seemed like a small price to pay for the opportunity to work with such an experienced avian practitioner. I called Dr. Petrak, introduced myself, and asked her permission to observe, or "shadow," her practice. I didn't realize at the time that Midge was as painfully shy as she was passionate about veterinary medicine in general and avian practice in particular. But she graciously agreed to my visits.

Every other week for the next eight months, I got into my car at 4 a.m. to drive to Boston and spend the day with Dr. Petrak. I would often return to Vermont as late as midnight. Although these days were long and tiring, I wouldn't have traded them for any other experience I've had in my career. The opportunity to work with Dr. Petrak, discuss cases with her, and watch her examination techniques—on the smallest finches to the largest macaws—was priceless. No lecture or textbook could have duplicated what I learned, and I became increasingly confident as I worked with birds in my own practice. I frequently consulted Dr. Petrak's book, using the excellent illustrations to educate both the birds' owners and myself.

In spite of this outstanding and groundbreaking text, it was a continuously troubling problem to try to keep abreast of the rapid expansion of knowledge in the new field. In 1980, however, a small group of veterinarians came together in Kalamazoo, Michigan and founded the Association of Avian Veterinarians (AAV), dedicated to the study and advancement of avian medicine. To further that aim, an annual scientific conference would be held, which would attract avian practitioners and researchers from around the country and eventually from around the world.

I learned of the AAV while working with Dr. Petrak, and I became a member immediately. In August of 1984, I attended the fifth annual meeting in Toronto, Ontario, and have gone to all except four annual meetings since that year. Having been a member of the American Veterinary Medical Association, the American Animal Hospital Association, the Rhode Island Veterinary Medical Association, and the Vermont Veterinary Medical Association, I had attended many scientific meetings since my graduation. However, from the first lecture and throughout the five-day meeting of AAV's Toronto conference, the level of knowledge and professional dedication of the speakers and attendees thrilled and electrified me.

At one AAV meeting I attended in Houston, Texas in 1988, we had a series of presentations on beak and feather disease—a terrible progressive condition first noted in cockatoos, in which new feathers come in deformed, and then fall out leaving the bird progressively more and more bald. In addition, the beak becomes misshapen and gangrenous so eventually the bird is unable to eat. The cause of this disease was unknown, there was no treatment, and it was 100 percent fatal. Because it seemed to be contagious, the most likely cause was thought to be a virus, but despite several years of intensive effort by many researchers, no one had yet been able to identify any causal organism, virus or otherwise. Beak and feather disease was a truly scary disease, especially when it was found to be contagious to species of birds other than cockatoos. This made every scrap of information, every observation about cases of the disease, extremely valuable to all veterinarians practicing avian medicine. The lecture room, needless to say, was packed.

Sitting next to me was a doctor whose badge identified him as Dr. Branson Ritchie from the University of Georgia. He was busy taking notes on other speakers' presentations, as would any other member of the audience. Imagine my surprise when the moderator announced that Dr. Branson Ritchie would give the next presentation— on identification of a virus thought to be the cause of beak and feather disease. The doctor sitting next me got up, went to the speaker's podium, and for the next thirty minutes, proceeded to outline his research, which had led to the identification of a virus that he (correctly) believed to be the cause of beak and feather disease. This was truly groundbreaking work, and the audience was completely absorbed as Dr. Ritchie narrated the thinking and methodology behind his research. This was a giant first step in diagnosing, understanding, and eventually, preventing the terrible disease. There were many questions and comments following this talk, and it was quite clear that Dr. Ritchie had the respect and admiration of all his colleagues, many of whom were also pioneers in their own right. After the question-and-answer period, Dr. Ritchie came down from the podium, and again, just like any other member of the audience, took his seat and began taking notes on the next speaker's presentation. Perhaps I am too easily impressed, but I felt quite honored to be sitting in the same room with people like Dr. Bran Ritchie.

Another memorable moment from the early days of the AAV was a presentation at an annual conference given by Dr. Greg Harrison, author and editor of the most comprehensive text in the field—Avian Medicine and Surgery. Dr. Harrison was another of the pioneer avian practitioners in the country. The subject of his talk was the introduction of a new, much safer anesthetic for use in avian surgery. Up until this time, most avian practitioners were using halothane, the inhalation anesthetic developed for use in humans by Dr. John Abajian.

Although this was an excellent anesthetic for people, and for dogs and cats, it was not ideal for birds for a number of reasons. Most birds have a rapid heart rate, a very high metabolic rate, and a much higher body temperature than dogs and cats—104 to 108 degrees Fahrenheit is normal for many parrot and songbird species. Under general anesthesia, reflexes are abolished, heart rate slows down, and body temperature decreases, all depending on the length of time the patient is anesthetized. The more rapid the recovery from anesthesia, the less physiological alteration occurs. Unfortunately, because of birds' unique respiratory systems, which are designed for efficiency during flight, recovery from halothane anesthesia is often dangerously prolonged, with sometimes-fatal results.

Dr. Harrison gave a brief talk on the merits of isoflurane—which is chemically related to halothane, but much faster acting—and detailed his experience with this anesthetic. Isoflurane was just starting to be used in human surgery and for horses, but it was Dr. Harrison and a few other pioneers who studied the characteristics of the drug and realized its potential as an avian anesthesia.

Next, Dr. Harrison brought out a portable anesthetic machine and an Amazon parrot. I happened to be sitting in the front row (I didn't want to miss a word at these conferences), so Dr. Harrison looked down at me and asked if I had a second hand on my watch. I said that I did, and he asked me to time how long it took this parrot to become anesthetized. He turned on the anesthesia machine and gently put the bird's head in a cone-shaped facemask of a type very commonly used in veterinary practice. In less than two minutes, the bird was sound asleep and breathing steadily and easily; this was half the time it would have required for induction with halothene. While continuing to discuss the merits of this anesthesia, Dr. Harrison allowed the parrot to remain anesthetized for three or four minutes.

Then came one of the most dramatic demonstrations I have ever seen. Dr. Harrison removed the mask from the bird's head and asked me to time the recovery from the anesthesia. In less than two minutes, the Amazon parrot was wide-awake, and in another minute, Dr. Harrison released the bird; we all witnessed a just-anesthetized parrot fly across the lecture hall in a perfectly coordinated manner. Dr. Harrison had certainly made his point about this new anesthetic. I would venture to say that most, if not all, avian surgeons today use either isoflurane or its newer "cousin" sevoflurane. Birds are one of the most challenging and fragile animals to anesthetize successfully and safely, and the use of isoflurane absolutely revolutionized avian surgery.

Dr. Ritchie's and Dr. Harrison's presentations were by no means the exception at the typical AAV annual conference. Two of the greatest honors I have had in my veterinary career have been being asked to be a member of the AAV's governing board for a three-year term, and presenting a case report at the thirty-first annual conference in front of my wonderful colleagues. The importance to avian medicine practitioners of having a regular and reliable forum to share new findings in the field cannot be overstated; considering how few bird owners were in the habit of using veterinary services at that time, it was crucial to be learning from each others' experiences.

My own experience with the owner of a certain little female cockatiel reinforced for me the fact that bird owners—like any other kind of pet owner—can defy the logic of economics with their devotion. This cockatiel story clearly answers the question about who would bring an inexpensive small bird to a veterinarian for tests, x-rays, and even surgery. For those not familiar with the species, cockatiels (not cockatoos) are small, perky, grayish birds with a standup feather crest on the top of their heads, and bright yellow and orange patches on their "cheeks." Breeders have succeeded in modifying their color patterns so that some have quite flashy and unique plumage. Cockatiels are not known for talking, but they are champion whistlers. I taught my cockatiel to whistle the opening bars to Beethoven's Symphony No. 5 and Tchaikovsky's 1812 Overture. They are very intelligent, sociable, and make excellent companions. They have one characteristic, however, which often causes them a lot of trouble: they are egg factories. The cockatiel hens lay loads of eggs, very frequently, and this is very hard on them because of the demand for calcium to make a good, hard eggshell. If the hen does not have enough calcium to give the developing egg a proper shell, she frequently cannot lay, or "pass," the egg. This condition is called egg-binding, and it can be life threatening because it exhausts the hen trying to lay the egg, and the egg puts pressure on nearby organs.

The other danger of a soft-shelled egg is that it may break inside the body, releasing yolk material into the surrounding tissues. This yolk material is very irritating and results in a severe inflammatory condition known as egg-yolk peritonitis, which can also be life threatening. In this scenario, the various organs in the body cavity become inflamed, as birds do not have a separate chest and abdomen—all their organs are in one space, called the coelomic cavity.

Because of these specific cockatiel worries, when I received an emergency call from Peg Dumas one evening telling me that her six-year-old female cockatiel, Isabelle, was acting lethargic and spending a lot of time down at the bottom of the cage, I told Peg to bring the bird in right away. As all bird owners should know, most birds dislike being on the ground for very long, and they will perch up higher unless they are too sick or weak to do so. It is a serious danger signal when a bird that normally uses a perch starts spending time at the bottom of the cage.

When any female cockatiel acts sick, one of my first suspicions is egg-binding, because it is so common. When I examined Isabelle, I could not feel an egg, but sometimes an egg can get stuck farther up in the coelom. To make sure, I took an x-ray of Isabelle, which did not show an egg, or at least not one with any shell; however, the film did show a very hazy coelomic cavity, which could be an indication of peritonitis. As I questioned Peg, she told me that Isabelle was a very prolific egg layer, but recently her eggs had seemed to be deformed and had soft shells. The more I thought about it, the more suspicious I was that Isabelle had egg-yolk peritonitis.

With egg-yolk peritonitis, there are generally two methods of treatment used: Give the hen antibiotics to prevent infection, and anti-inflammatory medication to control the reaction in the coelom and protect the intestinal tract, liver, and kidneys. This method, however, treats the symptoms and not the cause, and is often unsuccessful in saving the hen.

Surgically open the coelom and physically flush and remove the irritating yolk material. Provided the bird is not too sick, and is in the hands of a skilled avian surgeon, this method could provide much better results in resolving the problem.

Obviously, the surgical method is considerably more risky, and would be much more costly, especially since the nearest avian specialist surgeon was in Boston at Angell Animal Medical Center. (I was not about to attempt this particular procedure.) Peg Dumas was not a confident long-distance driver, and to my knowledge, she was not particularly affluent. But what was the lesson I'd learned at Warwick? Never prejudge? Peg Dumas put Isabelle in a carrier, got on a Vermont Transit bus, and went straight to Boston for Isabelle's surgery. Two days later, she was back with Isabelle, who seemed in fine condition; Peg had spent upwards of $1500 for her $50 cockatiel's treatment and care.

At the opposite end of the scale in my avian practice were my adventures with ratites—the family of large, flightless birds. This family includes ostriches, emus, and cassowaries. These birds are very powerful, can run at high speeds, and defend themselves with kicks from their long legs, the toes of which are armored with strong, sharp nails. Handling these creatures is definitely an art, and mistakes can result in severe injury to the handler.

The time I sutured up the eyelid of an ostrich at the Roger Williams Park Zoo while I was working at Warwick was an interesting experience, for sure. But that was a single bird, confined to a single stall in a barn. In the 80s, raising ostriches and emus (which are somewhat smaller than ostriches and easier to handle) became a popular agricultural enterprise, much like raising alpacas is today. The meat from these large birds was reportedly extremely low in cholesterol and very tasty, and the oil from their fat was supposed to rival olive oil for lightness and purity. Particularly in Texas, there were ranches with herds of hundreds of emus or ostriches. A proven breeding pair was worth up to $14,000!

As Vermont is such an agricultural state, it was a prime area for people willing to try their hand at breeding, raising, and marketing these formidable birds. Not surprisingly, the typical farm animal veterinary practitioner preferred to give them a "pass." Therefore, I was not very surprised when I received a phone call one morning from Bill Kipp of Bridport, Vermont. He introduced himself as having a "small herd" of about sixty emus. He needed to get health certificates for four of his birds because he was going to ship them to another state, and he needed identifying microchips implanted in several more birds. He'd heard that I "worked with birds," so it seemed perfectly reasonable to him that I would be happy to come to his farm and provide the services he needed.

As will become obvious, working with a six-foot tall emu that can run 20-25 miles an hour is a far cry from handling a twelve-ounce parrot or a one-ounce budgie. Although I had some reference material in my library and I had attended a few lectures on ratites at the AAV conferences, I felt far from skilled at working with these creatures, and I said as much to Mr. Kipp. Fortunately, he turned out to be quite knowledgeable about care and husbandry, and was an excellent emu handler. So I put on my farm coveralls, which I hadn't worn since veterinary school (I noticed they were a bit more "snug-fitting" than when I'd last put them on), and walked into the small pasture with Mr. Kipp and about fifteen young but large emus. They were very curious, and tried to nibble on anything dangling from our equipment kits or any loose clothing. I learned that the safe way to restrain them was to put one's arms around the long neck from behind and straddle the body, causing the bird to assume a sitting position. This wasn't too difficult when they were standing fairly still, but it was more like rodeo bulldogging when Mr. Kipp had to catch them "on the fly." Again, the trick was to never stand directly in front, because even the younger ones would kick if they didn't approve of being handled or examined. Once restrained, they seemed to be surprisingly agreeable to everything except having their head, eyes, ears, and mouth examined. All the while, the others crowded around us, trying to snatch syringes, gauze, and instruments—anything that caught their eye.

Because Bill Kipp had a sizable investment in his herd, he was willing to do almost any diagnostic procedure needed; for me, this made for a great learning experience. I had the opportunity to draw blood samples, do blood testing, perform x-rays on young birds that Mr. Kipp brought to my hospital, and perform some necropsies on birds that died of unknown causes. It is essential for a practitioner working with groups of animals, no matter what species, to perform necropsies, as the following story may help emphasize.

One sleet-filled February day I received an urgent call from Mr. Kipp. He was almost always cheerful and calm, so I could tell he was quite upset on the phone. It seemed that within the space of two days, four out of a group of twenty of his young adults had suddenly dropped dead, with no obvious warning signs. The others seemed healthy that morning, but so had the ones that died suddenly. This group of youngsters had all been housed in a barn for the last two weeks because of inclement weather. I didn't have to urge Bill to give permission for a necropsy; he asked if I could come down to the farm and examine the deceased emus because he was rightly worried that whatever killed the four he'd already lost would affect the rest of this group.

I finished my morning appointments and drove down to the Kipp farm. He had saved the bodies of two of the dead emus in a separate barn. Before I examined these emus, I asked Bill to take me to see the rest of the group. The minute we entered the barn where the rest of the group was being kept, my eyes began to smart because of a very strong ammonia odor coming from the damp straw bedding. I turned to Bill and asked him why he wasn't ventilating the barn—I could see four exhaust fans located along the walls of the bar, and they were not turning. Bill told me that there was a problem with the electrical supply to this barn, so the fans couldn't be used. He was concerned about the buildup of ammonia, but because of the ice right outside the barn, he was afraid to let the birds out for fear they might slip and fall. He realized, though, that the ammonia concentration was steadily getting worse.

Before we did anything else, we propped open the doors at each end of the barn—enough to let air circulate, but not enough to allow the birds to escape. I called my hospital and asked the receptionist to reschedule the afternoon appointments, and Bill and I removed all the straw from the barn—a job that took about two hours. When we were finished, the improvement in air quality in that barn was greatly improved. Only then did I start my examination of the deceased birds.

By this time I was becoming suspicious that the air quality in this barn had something to do with the deaths of the four emus. At a previous AAV meeting there had been several talks given on fungal infections in birds. One of the reports identified organic bedding as a common source of Aspergillus, a disease-causing, or "pathogenic," fungus. Bedding such as corncob was probably the worst offender in cases of caged birds, but wood shavings, straw, and bark (commonly used in reptile habitats) were also discussed. When I did the necropsy on the first bird, it didn't require a skilled pathologist to be fairly certain of the cause of death. Both of the bird's lungs were cobbled with raised white bumps, and so were the lungs of the second dead emu. I took tissue samples of the lungs for a pathologist to examine, but back at my hospital, I put some of the white material on a microscope slide and examined it. Sure enough, there were strands of fungus and spores everywhere. Conditions in

Steven B. Metz, d.v.m.

that barn must have been exactly optimal for what is called a fungal "bloom." The air had been full of infectious spores.

Six days later, the pathology report came back confirming the heavy infection by Aspergillus fungus, but by this time, the exhaust fans were working, the ice had been heavily sanded, and fortunately, Bill Kipp did not lose any more birds. His dilemma, however, was that the surviving birds had already been sold to an out-of-state emu farmer. Could he now, in good conscience, go through with the sale, knowing that although they appeared healthy at this point, they had been exposed to the same infection that had killed four others of the same group? Would the young emus remain healthy? For how long? Could these birds infect others on the new farm? All these questions he passed to me, and I felt it was my responsibility to help with his decisions. Here was yet another example of how, despite all the progress, all the research, all the expanding knowledge in avian medicine, we simply did not yet have many of the answers.

What I did know about Aspergillus infection was that we did not yet have a reliable antemortem (prior to death) test to identify carriers of the fungus, nor did we clearly understand whether or not a carrier bird could shed the fungus and infect others. Additionally, no vaccine against Aspergillus was available, and treatment of an infected patient was difficult and often unsuccessful. What we also knew about fungal infections was that a large number of infectious spores were usually necessary for disease to occur, and that good management practices were the best means of preventing the problem. The sales dilemma was eventually resolved by Bill Kipp agreeing to refund the purchase price of any bird that died or became ill due to aspergillosis.

Unfortunately for Mr. Kipp and the few others in Vermont who took a chance with the emu industry, no significant market developed for the meat or oil, and eventually emu and ostrich farming in Vermont became almost non-existent. My experience with the Kipp emus was exciting and stimulating—and there were other big-bird puzzles and adventures. Ratite medicine was in its infancy at this time, and any day, any case could produce totally new information.

There were two other areas of avian practice that were equally as challenging: raptors (owls and hawks), and small flock, or "backyard," poultry. The fascinating thing about my profession was that one moment I could be working with an eagle with a broken wing, and the next, a chicken with leg paralysis. What a contrast—to go from a completely wild creature to a common, domesticated one!

In this country, poultry means chickens and turkeys, and we usually think of the commercial poultry operation involving hundreds to thousands of birds raised under assembly-line conditions to produce eggs and meat. Because of this approach to poultry production, the biology and medicine of our friend, the chicken, has morphed into a unique and separate branch of avian medicine. It has resulted in a flock approach to diagnostics and medicine, as opposed to an individual patient approach. There are books, journals, and professional associations dedicated to those veterinarians who work almost exclusively in poultry medicine and related research. Much of our knowledge in other areas of avian medicine comes from the research and experience of these poultry specialists. In the United States, until recently, it has been quite rare for a veterinarian to work with both poultry and so-called "exotic" bird species, such as parrots, finches, and the ratite family.

In the past few years, there has been a great resurgence in small flock poultry—meaning anywhere from four or five hens to perhaps a dozen, rarely more. Even people living in some urban or suburban settings have chosen to keep chickens, usually for producing eggs. Raising small flocks of free-ranging chickens for natural or organic food production has become popular. The result of the small flock approach is that these chickens are treated quite a bit like pets. After all, a domestic chicken can have a distinctive and appealing personality. For example, when the owner of one such small flock went into the pen with her chickens and sat down, the hens would run to her and jump in her lap. The members of this small flock were all named after famous movie stars. The owner gave these names, she told me, only after careful observation of the individual personalities of each hen.

I freely admit to becoming particularly fond of some of my chicken patients. There was a black bantam hen named Rocket who had been attacked by the family dog, and had one wing badly broken, along with numerous lacerations—some of which were quite severe. Although the family had eight or nine other hens, there was no doubt in their minds that I should do everything possible to save Rocket. I put more than fifty stitches in the little hen (whom I put under general anesthesia), and I attempted to splint the broken wing. Rocket tolerated her splint with some reluctance, and scolded me every time I had to adjust it. After two or three follow-up visits, however, it became obvious that the injury to the bone and to the supporting soft tissue was so severe that this wing was not going to heal. In a dog or cat with this type of severe injury, the next step is amputation of the affected limb. I told Rocket's owners that I thought it was possible for Rocket to continue enjoying socializing with both her chicken and human families despite missing a wing. Without further hesitation, they asked me to perform the amputation surgery.

After her second major surgery, Rocket never looked back; she healed well. She was active and lived up to her name—soon she was zooming around her owners' mudroom and then the large pen and foraging area. Her personality became even more outgoing, and she actually became the official family greeter of visitors to the home.

Because I also took care of the family's dog that had been to blame for Rocket's injuries, I was able to keep track of Rocket for several years after her surgery. The owners never failed to let me know how glad they were to have made the decision to keep her, and that she had become a true member of the family.

I have had similar experiences with small flock ducks and geese, each species having their own requirements and problems. What sort of challenge might a duck present? How about using a facemask to try to anesthetize an animal that dives underwater to catch fish and can hold its breath for a long time? It is surprising how long it can take before such a patient is asleep enough to allow surgery. Fortunately, seminars, lectures, and textbooks on the medicine and surgery of poultry and waterfowl are becoming more common, and the pool of knowledge has expanded dramatically.

Less familiar is the medicine and surgery of hawks, owls, and other birds of prey. What can be done for these wildest of wild creatures, and why, you may ask? We share the same environment; we have created conditions that alter, and in many cases, endanger their lives. Thus it is a reasonable conclusion that we have a moral obligation to mitigate our impact on these magnificent bird species if we wish them to survive. A more practical answer is that these birds, along with other wild species, serve as monitors of our environment. We have only to think back to the example of the drastic reduction in population of the bald eagle and the peregrine falcon—the cheetah of the bird world. Back in the 1950s and 60s it was discovered that the widely used insecticide DDT was causing the eggshells of these birds to be too thin; the eggs were so fragile that they broke before the chicks could develop. Subsequently, it was discovered that DDT was being deposited in the bones of people around the world, even if DDT was not being used in that area! It was found that DDT dissolved in and evaporated with ground water, was carried great distances by wind currents, and was deposited in rainwater in all parts of the world. Similar to the coal miner's canary (which was used as a warning for high levels of methane gas present in mining tunnels), these birds of prey, being at the top of their food chain, were affected by the concentration of DDT. Once this was discovered, the use of the chemical was finally discontinued in 1972 in the U.S. and many other countries of the world. The bald eagle and peregrine falcon populations began—very slowly and gradually—to make a comeback; today both species have been removed from the endangered list.

However, it is still rare to see a bald eagle or peregrine falcon in Vermont. Thus, whenever there was an injured eagle, hawk, owl, or falcon in the northern part of the state, I was usually called on to help manage the situation. Shortly after coming to Vermont, I had become a member of the Vermont Institute of Natural Science (VINS)—a dedicated group of educators, researchers, and students of natural science headquartered in Woodstock. In addition to many other programs and services, they maintained a rehabilitation facility for injured birds of prey, and a housing facility for those birds too badly injured to be releasable back into the wild. This latter group of hawks and owls were used as educational birds for the statewide programs put on by VINS.

Because of my work with avian medicine and surgery, I was asked to become a member of the VINS Board of Directors, as well as the consulting veterinarian for their resident raptors and any injured birds of any species. As a result, one day I found myself working with a starving great blue heron who had waited too long to fly south, and the following day, I treated a loon that had unfortunately landed in a Sears parking lot in the rain because the wet asphalt looked like a pond.

I learned that loons' legs were located so far back on their body (to help propel them when diving for fish) that they were unable to walk on, or take off from, land. To help lift their heavy bodies, they needed a body of water large enough so they could run along the surface until they gained speed enough to fly. So the loon that picked the Sears parking lot, though fortunately uninjured, was stranded. When it was brought to me, I examined the bird, taking great care to avoid the extremely sharp, pointed bill. I found only a few minor scrapes. I wanted to make sure there were no unseen problems, however, so I sent one of my nurses out to a nearby bait shop to buy a small supply of large minnows. I put the loon in my bathtub, along with some minnows, and it quickly demonstrated that there was nothing wrong with its eyesight or appetite. As it was only a two-minute drive from there to the shores of Lake Champlain, I took this bird to the Shelburne boat access and put it in the water. Faster than the eye could see, the loon demonstrated its impressive diving skills—so completely that I began to wonder if it had just sunk to the bottom. But, no—

up the champion diver bobbed, about 75 yards out, and increased the distance between us every second. So much for the theory that wild creatures "sense when one is trying to help them."

As for the starving great blue heron—Vermont's tallest wading bird—this situation, I learned, was a regular fall occurrence. These avid fish- and frog-eating birds would stay near a pond or lake where there had been a reliable food supply all spring and summer, and they'd migrate south only when the colder weather made food scarce. If they waited too long, they became too weak to make the flight. Weak as they might be, they were still quite wild, and I learned that these and other species of wading birds such as bitterns and egrets, were extremely dangerous to handle. They would "play possum" when first captured, and then, using their extremely long, sharp-pointed bill and their very long necks, they could strike like a snake, frequently aiming for a person's eye (which must appear to them like a fish's or frog's eye).

Like many wild creatures, herons do not take kindly to captivity and usually refuse to eat, which only makes their weak condition worse. So they must be fed a blended liquid diet via stomach tube. Can you imagine slipping a tube all the way down that long neck? The dedicated and knowledgeable rehabilitators at VINS were often able to work miracles, however, and nothing was more satisfying than to be able to release a formerly sick or injured wild creature back into its natural habitat.

The release of a successfully rehabilitated bird was always a great event, and I frequently gathered with the VINS staff to mark the occasion. Unfortunately, the reason releases were celebrated with such ceremony was that it was not common to be successful in rehabilitating wild birds, especially raptors. The most frequent reason we received hawks, owls, and—very occasionally— eagles, was because of injuries, especially fractured wing bones. When this happened, the bird was grounded, enabling a Fish and Wildlife warden or good samaritan to capture the bird. Ideally, no one would be injured handling the hawk or owl (the sharp and extremely strong talons could inflict serious injury) and the bird would be quickly brought either directly to me, or to VINS. Somehow, even complete strangers to bird-handling never seemed to get hurt, but unfortunately, they often were so fascinated by these rare creatures that they kept the birds in their homes for a few days while a well-meaning "nurse" tried to feed the meat-eating birds bread and milk. This sometimes has tragic consequences, as in the case of a young couple who were thrilled when they found a beautiful snowy owl, too weak to fly, on the ground in their backyard.

These owls, normally inhabitants of the far north, occasionally migrate south when the rodent population in the Arctic and northern Canada is so decreased that the birds cannot sustain themselves. After migrating, the weakened birds find themselves in unfamiliar terrain and sometimes end up unable to hunt. This particular species is rather difficult to work with because they are normally very fearful, but the young couple tried to nurse the snowy owl back to health; however, the owl refused to eat the bread and milk and died after three days in the couple's home.

I should point out that although many people don't realize this, it requires federal and state licenses to handle, keep, and rehabilitate birds of prey and almost all wild birds, reptiles, and mammals. The purpose of these licenses is to insure that only knowledgeable, trained rehabilitators work with sick or injured birds and other wild species.

Back when I was describing some of my professors at the Ontario Veterinary College, I mentioned that Dr. Frank Milne, professor of equine surgery, told us that when repairing fractures in racehorses, "99-percent-success equals failure." At the time, I had little understanding or sympathy with that philosophy. In working with these avian athletes, however, I began to understand exactly what Dr. Milne meant to convey. Although it was not usually a matter of life or death if a horse couldn't race again (unless the owner decided otherwise), it was exactly that for hawks and owls. Falcons sometimes reach speeds of over 200 miles per hour in a dive (called a "stoop" by falconers), and other bird-hunting hawks—like the goshawk—have to be able to dodge in and around trees and bushes while flying at top speeds in order to eat. Any impairment of their flying ability usually means starvation. One of the most frustrating things about trying to repair a wing fracture in a bird of prey is that often the trauma causing the fracture (being hit by a car, flying into a window, hitting a power or telephone line) shatters the wing bones so badly that some of the pieces are actually missing. And even if all the bone is still there, the damage to the muscles, nerves, and blood vessels is so extensive that recovery is sometimes impossible.

Besides all those hurdles to overcome, most bird bones are constructed quite differently than mammalian bones. Most bones of flighted birds (not ratites) are hollow and relatively thin; they are designed to be lightweight. Therefore, fracture repair techniques used in mammals—such as inserting a stainless steel pin or rod into the central cavity or using a steel plate and screws to join the fractured pieces together—cannot be used in birds if they are to fly again.

After all, there is no marrow in flighted birds' "pneumatic" bones in which to sink pins or rods. And steel plates and screws are too heavy; the bones are simply too fragile. Special techniques, then, had to be developed to provide rigid, dependable, lightweight fixation and immobilization for fractured, hollow bird bones. One method I tried, as opportunity occurred, involved using Teflon rods instead of steel ones inside the bone, and fixing the rods in position with tiny steel pins perpendicular to the long axis of the bone, going through each side of the bone and the Teflon rod in the middle. The Teflon rods could be heat-sterilized, and were much lighter than steel. The very small fixation pins, called Kirschner wires, or "K-wires," were likewise almost negligible in weight. Additionally, with this method the Teflon rod did not have to extend the entire length of the bone as a steel rod does, thus reducing the weight even further.

Of course, no method can repair a broken bone if most of that bone is lying on some roadway, which is how VINS (and every other licensed rehabilitation or educational facility) obtained their captive raptors. If the hawk or owl could not fly normally, did not have full use and strength in its feet and talons, or if its vision was not normal, the bird could not survive in the wild. Then the choices were to find an educational facility in need of that particular species to house and care for the raptor, or humanely euthanize the unfortunate bird—as upsetting as that is to those of us who admire and care for these splendid creatures. Although it may seem contradictory, sometimes it is kinder not to sentence some of our wildlife species to a life in captivity.

When working with these patients, I always had to remind myself of their wild nature and unpredictability. In all my years of working with potentially dangerous patients—ranging from elephants and tigers to large snakes and even poisonous fish—it was a young injured red-tailed hawk that came closest to inflicting a severe injury, which would most likely have ended my career. Red-tailed hawks are one of the largest and most powerful of the soaring hawks in our area, and this young bird was a patient in my hospital with a bruised—not broken—wing. I was keeping him at my hospital so I could evaluate the progress of the wing. In retrospect, I would have been wiser to let an experienced rehabilitator with outdoor flight cages keep the hawk during his convalescence. Meanwhile, I fed the hawk killed mice (of which I kept a supply in my freezer), by holding the thawed mouse in a long pair of tongs and pushing it through the bars of the hospital compartment. After the second day, the red-tail would quickly grasp the mouse in his talons as I deposited it on the floor of the compartment. By the fourth day, he was anticipating being fed, and came to the front of the compartment as I approached. His wing was definitely getting better and he was able to flap it almost normally when I took him out of the compartment for his examination. Therefore, I decided to turn him over to one of the experienced rehabilitators in the Burlington area the next day to give him flight experience before releasing him.

Early the next morning, I admitted an elderly kitty who had kidney failure—one of the two or three most common causes of death in older cats—and carried her past the Red-tail's compartment to put her in a treatment compartment. I was in a hurry to get back to the upset owners in my exam room, so I wasn't thinking about the hawk as I approached his area on my return.

Normally, hawks and owls are not aggressive toward humans except when defending their nest areas or when trapped and defending themselves. But I had "trained" this young hawk to expect food when I came to his compartment. So as I came opposite to him, closer than usual (because my mind was on the elderly, sick cat and the owners), he reached out in a lightning-fast snatch through the bars of the compartment door and sunk only one (fortunately) of his inch-and-a-quarter long, razor-sharp talons into my face, just a little below my left eye. My immediate reflex, of course, was to jerk my head backward—which may well have saved my eye. Had the red-tail gotten a grip with all four of his immensely strong talons, at the very least I would likely have lost a sizable piece of both my face and eye.

As I leaned back against the opposite wall and tried to calm myself down, my memory flashed back to Miss Claudia Schmidt, my seventh grade science teacher who had introduced me to the world of birds. I couldn't help it—I murmured, "We've come a long way from Forest Park bird walks, haven't we, Miss Schmidt?"

chapter ten

Not Your Average Companion

If asked what one experience was the "crown jewel" of my career as a veterinarian, I would reply without hesitation, "The tiger."

One Saturday afternoon in late May, I had finished my appointments for the day, my technicians had left, and I was getting ready to close the hospital. I hoped to be able to relax and enjoy the rest of the weekend with my family. Just as I was walking out the door, the phone rang. I debated in my head whether to answer it or let the answering service take the call. I had repeatedly given the answering service strict instructions that if there was any doubt at all whether a caller had a true emergency, they were to call me; therefore, I felt fairly certain I would end up taking this call one way or another. So, I picked up the phone and answered, "Shelburne Veterinary Hospital, Dr. Metz speaking."

The caller asked, "Are you the vet that works with wild animals?" I cautiously admitted that I did often treat non-domestic species. The caller continued, "I'm calling from the fairgrounds, and I have a really sick tiger." Now, over the years, some of my relatives and friends have tried to play tricks on me by challenging me to come treat their elephant, their wolf, their snake, or their tiger, and so I replied to this caller, "Sure you have a sick tiger, and I'm really President George Washington."

Evidently the caller had met with skepticism before, so he assured me, "No, really, I'm up here with the Shriners' Circus, and one of my cats is really sick. I'm afraid she may not make it. Can you please come?" I was immediately convinced that this was not a joke. I told the caller I would be out within the hour, packed everything I could think of into my house call bag, and drove out to the fairgrounds in Essex Junction, a neighboring community to Burlington. As I drove, I worried to myself: What the devil do I know about large felines, their diseases and treatments, medications to use, dosages … ? I was still thinking about these questions when I arrived at the fairgrounds and was met at the gate by Mr. Alan Gold and his helper, Holly. They led me directly to the area where their circus wagons were parked, and in one large wagon was a huge female Bengal tiger. Instead of being up, alert, and walking around in the wagon as were the other cats, this tiger was stretched out and nearly motionless. Not even her ears twitched when I walked up to the cage. Alan Gold had not exaggerated. She was indeed a very sick cat.

I turned to Alan and said, "Well, bring your squeeze cage over and I'll examine her."

"Don't have a squeeze cage," he replied.

A squeeze cage is a set of strong bars on railings, which is placed inside the cage or wagon; the bars can be cranked to confine the cat to a narrow space against the side of the cage. This prevents the big cat from having the would-be examiner for breakfast! A squeeze cage is considered by most circus and zoo veterinarians to be an absolutely essential piece of equipment for handling large, dangerous animals of all types.

After I digested the fact of no squeeze cage, I said (exact wording not guaranteed), "Holy Smoke! How the dickens am I supposed to examine her? She's much too sick to anesthetize or even sedate." Without waiting for an answer, I retrieved a large rectal thermometer intended for horses from my bag, lubricated it, and—carefully watching for the cat's reaction—reached through the bars of the cage and inserted the thermometer into the appropriate opening. Princess—that was her name— "grumbled" a bit but fortunately did not move. When I removed the thermometer and read it, I noted that her temperature was 101.5 degrees Fahrenheit.

I was not sure of the normal rectal temperature of a tiger. This reading would have been well within normal range of a domestic house cat, but I knew that, metabolically, larger animals tend to have significantly lower body temperatures than small animals. For example, the normal temperature for a horse is about 99.5, while that of a mouse is closer to 104. Taking this into consideration, I felt that a temperature of 101.5 probably indicated a fever in this large cat. I showed the thermometer to Alan and Holly, and said, "I really need to examine her, but I don't see how I can."

"What do you want to look at?" asked Alan.

"I want to look at her mucus membranes—for example the upper, white part of her eye, but I don't suppose that's possible," I answered.

Without a word, Alan Gold climbed into that circus wagon, went up to the tiger's face, and speaking soothingly to her, lifted up her upper eyelid. After I swallowed and closed my dropped jaw, I moved closer, and noted that the white of Princess's eye seemed to be tinged with a yellowish color.

"What else do you want to see?"

"I—well—I'd like to see the color of her gums, but I'm sure that's quite impossible," I said. Using the word "dangerous" seemed absurd under the present circumstances.

No sooner had I pronounced the word "impossible" than Alan reached his bare hand across the tiger's muzzle and lifted her upper lip, revealing huge fangs (nothing diminutive about the rest of her dentition, either) and obviously yellow-colored gum tissue.

All this time, while Alan Gold—completely unprotected in any way—had his hands and body inches from this tiger's teeth and claws, I was standing outside the wagon with my eyes bugged out and jaw dropped. Everything I had read and learned about handling wild species, not to mention every natural instinct, shouted that handling an adult tiger in this manner was insanity. I felt like an idiot standing outside the wagon while Alan was poking at Princess's eyes and putting his hands in her mouth.

The next step in any meaningful examination was to listen with a stethoscope to the patient's heart and lungs, which I could not do from outside the wagon. I looked at Alan and asked, "What do you think about me coming into the wagon and putting a stethoscope on her chest?"

"Come on in," he said. "I won't let anything happen."

It would be difficult to say who was more irrational: Alan Gold, for handling this immensely powerful wild creature in such a manner and for making the completely ridiculous statement suggesting he could stop the tiger should she decide we had outworn our welcome, or me, for climbing into that circus wagon.

To make matters even more interesting, the stethoscope I was using at the time had tubing only fourteen inches long, allowing a total distance of about twenty inches between my face and the tiger's shoulder and front legs. Nevertheless, with a shaky hand, I placed the head of the stethoscope firmly against the tiger's rib cage just behind her left front leg, then on the right side (she was so big that I had to walk around her rear), and listened. Because I had never before listened to a big cat's heart or breathing sounds, I had, once again, to use the parameters of horse cardiology and respiration. Irregular heart rhythm and wheezing sounds are essentially the same throughout the animal kingdom, however, so I wasn't completely at a loss for assessment. Fortunately, I heard no abnormalities, either with the heart or with respiration.

The next step in a complete examination was to feel, or "palpate," the tiger's abdomen. This involved firmly pressing against different areas on both sides of her belly. I told Alan what I wanted to do.

"Go ahead, she seems relaxed," he said.

But at my first firm press just behind her rib cage, she lifted her head and tried to look around. I didn't wait for comments from Alan; I exited the wagon promptly! Alan followed a moment later, after stroking the big cat's head.

"What do you think, Doc?" he asked.

"I think the next step is to take a blood sample," I replied. "The whites of her eyes and her gums have a yellowish color to them—she's jaundiced. The most common cause of jaundice is a liver problem, and given her fever, I suspect it might be hepatitis. Can you think how she may have picked up an infection?"

"Could spoiled meat cause it? On our last stop farther south, I bought some beef that just didn't smell right."

"Yes. Definitely," I said. "With a blood sample, we can be pretty sure what we're dealing with."

Now I'd really put my foot in it. A blood sample was needed for a diagnosis, but how in heck was I to get the sample from an awake tiger? I didn't care how many Alan Golds were between Princess's face and me. I was not going to walk up to her and put a needle in her front leg—one common site for drawing blood from a domestic dog or cat. I was not even going to go into the wagon and put a needle in her back leg.

Again, as happened when I was asked to determine a horse's age during the New York State licensing examination, there came a vivid flashback. In Dr. J.Y. Henderson's book Circus Doctor, Dr. Henderson tells of the difficulty in getting blood samples from big cats. To solve this problem, he performed a detailed necropsy on an elderly circus lion that had died from unknown causes—specifically looking, not only for the cause of death, but for a large vein near the surface of the cat's skin, a vein which would be accessible in an unanesthetized animal. In spite of the fact that I hadn't read the book in over twenty years, I remembered that he had located such an accessible vein running along the underside of the tail. Perfect! All we had to do was to hold the tail still enough, and I had to be able to "hit" the vein, preferably without unduly aggravating Princess.

A circus, especially when on the road, functions like a close-knit family, and by this time, we had a small gathering of other circus performers around Princess's wagon. Alan seemed a bit skeptical about the blood sample. He didn't know me or my competence, and Princess was the "star" of his performance, leaping through a hoop of fire on command. But having little choice, he asked four of the huskiest onlookers to help, and he slipped a rope around the cat's tail, pulling it out through the bars of the wagon so that all five people were holding the tail. Princess growled (it sounded like thunder) and tried to turn around. I quickly put a tourniquet around the tail to make the vein stand out more prominently, and—wonder of wonders—I hit the vein first try and drew a perfect blood sample, just as if I'd done it a hundred times! We were all surprised at how smoothly it went. I got several congratulations of "Nice going, Doc," from the circus folk.

Now I had to get the blood sample analyzed, but it was Saturday afternoon, and I had a really sick patient. The analysis should not wait until I could send it overnight by air to my regular veterinary laboratory on Monday. Anticipating the diagnosis, I started treatment for the presumed bacterial hepatitis by reaching through the bars and administering a horse-sized injection of amoxicillin and another of vitamin B complex in the muscle of a hind leg. Princess didn't like it, but evidently was too weak to protest with any enthusiasm. Then I quickly left the fairgrounds, telling Alan I would be back in the early evening to check on Princess. I drove straight to the Medical Center Hospital in Burlington, and took the sample to the laboratory.

The Medical Center Laboratory was not doing veterinary samples at this point, so I expected some resistance when I asked them to do a non-human analysis. But I spoke to the technician on duty, explained the situation, and told her exactly what tests I needed. In fact, she was quite excited about doing blood analysis for a sick tiger, but warned me that her lab had no idea what results were normal; I would be on my own in the interpretation of these results. I thanked her, left the sample, then drove back to my hospital, where I hoped my library would be of some help with the blood results. (This was before Google, or any other computerized pool of information.) I didn't find a listing of normal tiger blood values anywhere in my books or journals, but I did find a reference to pioneering work in large cat medicine being done at the Cincinnati Zoo. I immediately picked up the phone and put in a call to the chief veterinarian there. The veterinarian, whose name I cannot recall, was not on the premises. I expected that—it was a Saturday afternoon, after all—but I reasoned that somewhere on or in the zoo's veterinary office, there would be a phone number to call in case of emergency. I next called the zoo's security police, told them that I had an emergency situation, and asked them to give me the emergency number. As I expected, they would not give this number out to just anyone who called. I explained that I was a veterinarian in Vermont, that I had a really sick tiger on my hands, and that their veterinarian was a nationally recognized authority on tigers. I think it was the fact that I knew about their veterinarian, of whom they were obviously proud, that convinced them. Over the next hour, they tracked down the chief veterinarian of the Cincinnati Zoo, and soon after that I received a phone call from this wonderful colleague.

After listening to my description of the physical exam, the jaundice, fever, and history of ingestion of possibly spoiled meat, he agreed that hepatitis should be at the top of the list of possible diagnoses. He gave me some suggested doses of the medications I had already started, and encouraged me to continue treatment. He also was able to give me some normal values for the blood tests I had ordered from the lab. For at least the third time in my career, I had been "rescued" by an outstanding member of my profession.

Three hours after I left the sample with them, the Medical Center laboratory had the results of the blood tests. They revealed an elevated white blood cell count, which indicates an infection, and elevated liver enzymes and very high levels of serum bilirubin, or bile, which indicates liver involvement. I went back to the fairgrounds about seven o'clock that evening—I certainly didn't want to treat Princess in the dark—took her temperature, and gave her a second set of injections. Her temperature was down a half a degree to 101.0, but she was still lethargic and barely raised her head when I gave her the medication.

I told Alan and Holly about the blood results and about the conversation I'd had with the Cincinnati Zoo veterinarian. By now, Alan had thawed out considerably and was feeling more optimistic about Princess's chances for recovery. He told me that he'd had some less-than-satisfactory experiences with veterinary care as he traveled around the country, and that when he had to call a veterinarian, he never knew whether he was getting someone who really knew about zoo animal medicine. In turn, I told him that my experience with big cats had been limited to my one treatment of the leopard chin abscess in Rhode Island, but that I had spent two days as a young boy with Dr. Henderson at Ringling Brothers and had read his book over and over. I also said that I had been lucky to spot the jaundice in Princess's eye-whites and gums; otherwise, the diagnosis would not have been as clear. I promised Alan that I would treat his tiger twice daily until it was clear that she either was or was not getting better and that I would not hesitate to speak with the Cincinnati Zoo veterinarian as many times as necessary.

The next morning I went out to the fairgrounds to find a different tiger in the circus wagon. Princess was up, walking—slowly, but walking—and Alan, who was thrilled by the improvement, told me that she had seemed interested in eating, but that he hadn't wanted to feed her until I came. It was much more difficult to take Princess's temperature this time, but when I did get the reading, it was down to 99.8. By letting her nibble some cooked beef (from his bare hands!), Alan distracted her enough so I could get the injections into her. From this point on, Princess continued to get stronger and more active. Taking her temperature was out of the question and her injections became almost impossible. I switched to oral medications hidden in her food, which worked well, as she had regained her appetite. I continued to visit her twice a day for the next five days to make sure she continued her recovery.

Three days before the circus' opening day, Alan asked me if I thought Princess could perform. I was dubious because she had been so seriously ill.

"You'll have to be the judge of her strength," I told him, "but we can get an idea of how her system is recovering from the liver infection by analyzing another blood sample."

Alan agreed. But we had quite a different patient on our hands this time. As much as I hated to put her through the stress, it took four people to rope Princess's front end to the bars of the wagon, and another four to restrain her tail. Now, for the first time, I came to understand the astounding power and ferocity of this big cat. I do not exaggerate one bit when I say that the ground under my feet shook with her roars. I will never forget the sound. The raw power of this animal—into whose cage I had climbed just a few days ago, and whom I had been injecting twice daily—was stunning. Because Princess was struggling, I was only able to get a very small blood sample this time, but I knew that the Medical Center laboratory was accustomed to having a spare amount of the sample in case there was a problem with the analysis. In fact, they required an extra amount or they would reject the sample with the notation "QNS," which meant "quantity not sufficient." I was sure this was the treatment this small sample would receive unless I intervened. When I arrived at the laboratory, I asked to speak to the head technician. When an energetic young lady came to the front counter, I held up the vial containing Princess's blood and said, "This is a sample from a 600-pound Bengal tiger, and there isn't going to be any more available. So let's figure out how we can get the results I need from this small sample. Q-N-S just cannot happen."

Once she understood the situation, I saw why she was the head technician. She immediately called together the two technicians who would actually be performing the analysis and we discussed what tests to prioritize if we didn't have enough blood to do a complete analysis. Between the three technicians, they decided to use the same techniques that would be used to analyze a blood sample from a newborn baby, which obviously requires a much smaller amount of blood than normal. In the end, due to the skill and care of the laboratory team, I was able to get all the test results I needed.

The results confirmed that Princess's system was indeed responding to the medications. Her white blood cell count was down, and her liver enzymes were down closer to the normal range too. When I discussed these results with Alan, he decided to have Princess in the ring for the performance, but not to have her jump through a hoop of fire from one pedestal to another, which was the grand finale of his act. The trick required great strength and agility, and it was an extremely difficult thing to teach a cat to do because animals instinctively avoid fire. If Princess's aim was even slightly off or she misjudged her landing, she could be severely burned or injured. I agreed with Alan's decision, and asked him if my family and I could attend the performance and sit "close to the action." He said that he and Holly were counting on it and had reserved seats for us in the front row of the grandstand.

Meanwhile, other circus people had started to warm up to "the Doc" during the course of my twice daily visits, and the day after I took the second blood sample from Princess, the elephant trainer came over to see me. He had recently rescued (or liberated, depending on your opinion of zoos) an elderly female elephant from a zoo across the Canadian border in Granby, Quebec. This elephant was not in very good physical condition, and the trainer was trying to improve her health with daily injections of vitamin B12. The problem was that after a few of these injections, the elephant was becoming "needle-shy," and would not stand still for the trainer.

"What size needle are you using?" I asked him.

He showed me a 16-gauge needle (the smaller the number, the larger the needle) that he'd purchased from a farm animal veterinarian in Quebec. For comparison, I had been using 22-gauge needles for Princess's injections, a common size for "small animal" practitioners to use when giving injections. The elephant trainer's 16-gauge needles looked like pipes compared to the 22-gauges I had been using.

"Holy cow!" I said. "If someone came at me with a needle of that size, I'd run like hell."

Because this elephant had become needle-shy, I decided to use an even smaller, 25-gauge needle—the size I often use when giving injections to my bird species patients. When I showed these very small needles to the trainer, he

154   S t e v e n   B .   M e t z ,   d . v . m .

laughed and said, "You're dealing with an elephant, here, Doc. You won't even be able to get that through her skin."

I admit to having never before given an injection to an elephant, but I remembered reading in Circus Doctor that "elephants have tender skin." So I drew up the vitamin B12 solution into my syringe, fitted a 25-gauge needle to it, and said to the elephant trainer, "If you could just stand by her head."

I walked up to the elephant's shoulder, reached up, clapped her firmly two or three times with the palm of my hand, then with the same motion, inserted the needle through the skin, injected the vitamin solution and withdrew the needle. She didn't so much as a twitch! The expression on that elephant trainer's face was priceless; he had been working with elephants far longer than I had been a veterinary practitioner, and I had just done something that he firmly believed was impossible. I left him a supply of the small needles and went back to the hospital, but even before I drove away, I saw him with a crowd of circus workers around him. He was holding up one of the tiny needles and gesturing toward his elephant.

The evening of the opening circus performance, Connie and I went to the seats Alan had reserved for us in the grandstand at the fairgrounds. Holly came out to make sure we were there and waved. Shortly, the circus parade—featuring all the animals except Alan's cats, but including the elderly elephant—began at the opposite side of the circular track. When the leading horses with their very glamorous rider drew opposite to our seats, the parade stopped, the glamorous lady rider jumped off her horse holding a large lei of colorful flowers, climbed into the grandstand, and put the flowers over my head and around my neck. At the same time, to my great embarrassment, the public address announcer asked me to stand and introduced me as the area veterinarian "who had saved two of the most valuable performers in the circus." There was a round of applause from the audience, and then the performance began.

The first act was "Alan Gold and his Educated Felines," and before he began his act, he pointed to Princess sitting impressively on her pedestal and waved to me. I grinned and waved back.

At that moment I felt that I had honored the memory of the "Circus Doctor," Dr. J.Y. Henderson, who had been an example and an inspiration to me from the time I first knew I wanted a career in veterinary medicine.

In recent years, for various reasons, big cat and elephant acts have become rare, except in large circuses, but that did not end my association with either species. About five years after the Shriners' Circus, my next "big cat adventure" began with a phone call from an assistant chief of police in a community not far from Burlington. I knew this gentleman, because he had previously owned a beautiful Doberman pinscher, and I had a reputation for being particularly fond of the breed. His name has been changed to protect his privacy. His voice on the other end of the line said, "Dr. Metz, this is David Dubois, and I'm in a very difficult situation. I urgently need your help."

The situation was that Mr. Dubois had recently been to Florida and had purchased a cougar kitten—a mountain lion, cougar, puma, whatever one chose to call it—on the "black market." As we will see, one can purchase almost any creature on the black market. At the time, the kitten had been only six or seven weeks old and was quite cute. Mr. Dubois felt sure he could raise this kitten successfully and safely in his home, but when the kitten began to shred and destroy his home only two months later, he realized he had made a terrible mistake. To his credit, once he came to this realization, Mr. Dubois had diligently made phone calls until he found a wild animal farm in New Hampshire that agreed to take the young cougar provided a veterinarian had examined the cat and it had the required vaccinations. Apparently, that was where I came in. Mr. Dubois had been at the Shriners' Circus and thought that if I could care for an adult tiger, I could certainly help with a cougar kitten.

"How big is the 'kitten' now?" I asked.

"Just four months old," was the evasive reply. I felt sure that David had a good reason for not answering the size question. We made an appointment for him to bring the cougar in when no other patients would be in the reception or examination rooms.

I happened to be in the rear area of the hospital when David and his cougar kitten arrived, and so I didn't get a glimpse of them at first. But I did see my technician Alison emerge from the examination room with a wide-eyed and apprehensive expression. As I was getting ready to go into the exam room, she warned me, "He's pretty big and pretty rambunctious." I prepared the needed vaccines in advance, handed the loaded syringes to Alison, took a deep breath, and said to her, "Follow me."

I was carrying a sheaf of forms as I entered the room. The next thing I knew, I saw a gigantic paw coming at me, and I was knocked to the floor by a buff-colored cannonball hitting me squarely in the chest. The cougar "kitten" (I estimated his weight at 25 to 30 pounds) was feeling playful. As we were rolling around on the floor "playing," I gasped to Alison, "Quick, hand me the syringes." I managed to extricate my arm from the huge paws wrapped around it, take the syringes one after the other, and administer the injections—it didn't matter where they landed (as long as they were somewhere on the "kitten's" body). The cougar seemed to regard the injections as just another form of play, and continued to drag me around the floor by my sleeve, while shaking my arm to see if he could detach it.

I did get a fairly good look at his teeth (large and white), his skin, his feet (very close up, and fortunately with retracted claws), eyes and nose, but that was the extent of the physical exam. I'm sure he would have shredded or swallowed my stethoscope had I attempted to listen to his heart and lungs. In spite of this abbreviated examination and judging by the way he was dragging an object seven times his body weight around the room, it was hard to imagine any physical problems with this ball of muscular dynamite. Although it only took about two minutes—it seemed much longer—as David tried to snap a leash to the harness the kitten was wearing. Finally, he was successful, and I staggered to my feet. I felt as if I'd just gone three rounds with a bulldozer! I signed all the necessary forms and sent David Dubois and his cougar "kitten" on their way.

Although all three of my close encounters with members of the "big cat family" (the leopard in Rhode Island, the tiger named Princess, and this cougar) included moments of actual terror, I was thrilled, in retrospect, to have had these experiences. They were certainly, to say the least, uncharacteristic in the career of the typical companion animal veterinary practitioner. Fortunately or unfortunately, the cougar was the last large cat I have been called upon to examine or treat thus far. Likewise, my experience with elephants has had its "last hurrah" with the Big Apple Circus matriarch, Anna Mae—a highly educated and much loved performer.

The calls always seemed to come on a Saturday. This time, when the caller identified himself as with the Big Apple Circus and said that he had an elephant with an infected eye, I didn't claim to be President George Washington. The circus was camped at the Shelburne Museum grounds just three miles from my hospital. Taking everything I could think of for an eye exam and treatment, I drove into the circus encampment fifteen minutes later. The elephant trainer, who was a man of few words, gestured towards a large female Indian elephant standing under a giant tent. I cautiously walked over close to her, and noticed that she was squinting with one eye, and there was a discharge dribbling down her cheek. Elephant eyes are surprisingly small when you consider the size of the head into which they are set. In order to examine her eyes I was going to need a tall stepladder. I turned to the trainer to ask for the ladder that I rea-

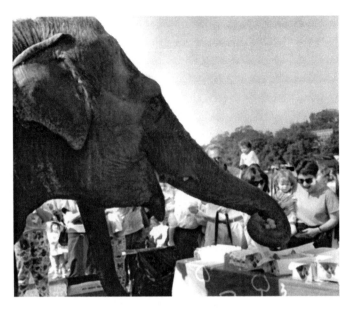

Anna Mae was the elephant matriarch of the Big Apple circus.

soned he must have handy. Instead, he walked up to this very large creature and commanded, "Anna Mae, down," just as I would direct a trained dog. And sure enough, just like a house dog, Anna Mae knelt down, which put her eye at just about the level of my eye as I stood on tiptoe. With the trainer standing beside me at her head, I gently and carefully spread her eyelids open (it took all the strength in my fingers) so I could see her eye. Then, using a pinpoint light and an ophthalmoscope, I examined the surface of the eye—the cornea, the pupil, and the tissue surrounding the eye called the conjunctiva. Putting my eye right next to Anna Mae's was another truly unique experience. Just as Alan Gold, the tiger trainer, would have been completely helpless to prevent his tiger from being as destructive to us both as she chose, this elephant trainer obviously could have done nothing to prevent his elephant from swatting us both like a couple of bothersome fleas had she been so inclined.

In part, that is why I didn't put special drops of sterile dye (fluorescein) into her eye to make sure she did not have a scratch on the cornea, a procedure that would have required considerable cooperation from Anna Mae. I could see no obvious evidence of any problem with the eye itself, however the tissues around the eye were obviously very irritated. It is true I had never specifically studied the elephant eye, but in general, the anatomy is the same as the eye of a dog, horse, or human—but very different, by the way, from the avian, reptilian, or fish eye. Here again, an amazing veterinary education (plus overcoming some shaky nerves) allowed me to perform a meaningful examination and to recognize signs of disease common throughout the world of mammalian eyes. Anna Mae had conjunctivitis, and the treatment was the same, whether treating an elephant or a pet mouse.

I showed the taciturn trainer how to apply antibiotic ointment to his elephant's eye, left him several tubes of ointment (ophthalmic medication manufacturers did not have elephants in mind) and promised to check on Anna Mae in two days. He said, "Thanks," then turned back to his elephant and had a quiet, private conversation with her; he was obviously much more interested in speaking with her than with me. But I knew I was gaining approval from the trainer when, on my return visit two days later, he extended his hand and said, "She's much better, thanks very much, Doc." Much to my pleasant surprise, he then invited me to come to the following Saturday's performance and watch from behind the scenes, which I did.

In recent times, circuses, particularly smaller traveling ones that feature trained animal acts (including dogs and horses), have been harshly criticized for the inhumane treatment of the animals involved. I am sure this criticism is merited in many cases—but not in every case. It so happens that the three circuses with which I have been involved merit the opposite reaction. No one could have been more involved with their animals than Anna Mae's trainer or Alan Gold—whom I later visited in Quebec and found bringing up his daughter and a young tiger cub together. Concern for their animals was uppermost in these men's minds, and although neither trainer was particularly affluent, there was absolutely no question but that I should do anything and everything to help their charges. It could be argued that these animals were the trainers' bread and butter. It was my strong feeling, however, that the relationship between Anna Mae and her trainer, and between Princess and Alan, was far deeper than mere dollars and cents.

The more I was among circus people, the more I realized they were a unique group—a family in every sense. They traveled with their children and educated them on the road, between practices and performances, and they were forced to trust unknown doctors, veterinarians, and other professional people for needed services. I hereby enter a plea for those of us who love and respect animals not to automatically condemn what we may not understand.

Nothing can illustrate the diversity of the so-called "exotics" part of my practice better than switching from tigers and elephants to ... goldfish. Not possible, you say? Who in the world would seek veterinary care for an individual goldfish—not a whole pond full or even an aquarium, but one fish that had been in the family for several years? That is exactly what a somewhat shame-faced middle-aged gentleman came to my front desk to ask me to do one morning. This particular goldfish had a lump on its side that was gradually getting larger; it was upsetting the fish's balance while swimming. The owner wanted to know if I'd ever done surgery on a fish before. I said that I had not, but that if the growth did not involve any internal organs and was just on the surface of the skin, I might be able to remove it. I advised him that there was risk involved, but he didn't hesitate—nor did he ask the cost of the surgery—and he agreed to bring the fish in the next morning.

That evening I reviewed the literature on surgery of fish using the indispensable, computerized Veterinary Information Network, started by Dr. Paul Pion and another of his colleagues. (I had joined the network in 1994 when it was in its infancy; present membership is approximately 47,000.) I learned that I did not have the medication commonly used to anesthetize fish, so I wanted to try bubbling isoflurane—the same general anesthetic I would use on a dog or a bird—through the water of a shallow pan in which I planned to perform the surgery. The most important considerations, as they are with any surgery on any species, was to make sure our patient continued to breathe steadily and was properly anesthetized so as to be free from pain. What was unique to this surgery was that fish have a coating of clear mucus over their scales, which helps to protect them from infections and parasites, and it was very important not to damage or dry out this "slime coat" during the surgery.

The next morning, I placed the six-inch common goldfish (not one of the fancy varieties) in a pan of water and let a mixture of isoflurane anesthetic and oxygen bubble into the water. It worked like a charm! Inside of ninety seconds, the goldfish turned on its side and floated to the top of the pan—normally this would be cause for great alarm, except that the gills continued to move in normal rhythm and rate. This was admittedly a crude and incomplete way to monitor the effects and depth of anesthesia, but it was all we had. My team and I supplied lots of extra oxygen to the water and we kept the water temperature warmer than normal.

Wearing latex surgical gloves so as not to damage the scales, and using a conventional surgical scalpel, I quickly sliced off the growth, about the size of a

S t e v e n   B .   M e t z ,   d . v . m .

penny, from the fish's side. There was a small amount of bleeding, which I had a little trouble stopping until I gently elevated just the surgical area above the surface of the water and used chemical cautery. Within seconds of turning off the isoflurane, the goldfish righted itself and started to swim around the pan in a normal manner.

We watched the fish for about an hour post-surgically to make sure there was no further bleeding and no "hangover" from the anesthesia, and then we sent it home with a very happy owner. I don't remember what the charges were for this "sophisticated" surgery, but I do recall that I got quite a chuckle out of being able to say that I had treated everything from elephants and tigers, to mice and fish. The growth on the goldfish turned out to be a "granuloma," a growth usually caused by infection, inflammation, or a foreign body. Unfortunately, I lost track of the little creature, so I cannot report on the long-term effects of the surgery.

In recent years, as knowledge has increased and technology improved, saltwater aquariums have become more popular. They are definitely more labor-intensive than the more familiar fresh water setups and require considerable skill to maintain. Saltwater fish are often very expensive, especially the more exotic species. Thus it was no surprise when I received a call from a gentleman in a nearby community inquiring if I had any experience with saltwater fish. I answered that I had not (although as a grade and high school student, I had kept and bred several species of freshwater tropical fish). Because of this early experience with tropical freshwater fish, I was familiar with the condition known as "fin rot," with which one of this gentleman's most exotic fish was infected. There are several different causes of fin rot, I knew, and the quickest way to diagnose the problem was to take a fin biopsy—that is, to snip off a small piece of the affected fin and have it examined microscopically by a knowledgeable pathologist. This is usually a quick and easy procedure, not requiring anesthesia, and I told this fish-owner about it.

"What species of fish are we talking about?" I inquired.

"A lionfish," was the answer.

For those who may not be familiar with saltwater fish, I should describe the lionfish as a striped creature, flattened from side to side (not top to bottom like a flounder or halibut), and with poisonous spiny fins sticking out in all directions like porcupine quills. To make things more exciting, this fish can often be quite aggressive and will lunge at anything it perceives as a nearby threat. A sting from one of these spines, I'm told, is very painful; I had to get my biopsy

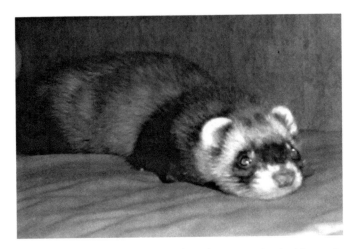

For some time, ferrets like Ms. Sable (above) were considered wild animals and were illegal to keep as pets.

specimen from one of these spines.

Because this fish was not easy to handle, I would have to do the biopsy as a house call, without removing the fish from the aquarium. As it turned out, it was not that difficult. I trapped the fish against the side of the aquarium with a net and wore thick gloves hoping to prevent a sting. I snipped off a piece of fin between lunges of the fish, carefully grasped the specimen with a pair of thumb forceps, placed it in preservative, and shipped it to the pathologist I used—Dr. Drury Reavill, out in California, who happens to have a particular interest in the biology and medicine of fish. She identified the problem as being a fungal infection and the owner, to whom I was quite content to leave the task of treatment, successfully restored the fins of his lionfish to their former "splendor." In spite of the fact that this fish's body was only the size of the palm of my hand, and that a sting, if it had occurred, would most likely only have been painful rather than dangerous, I would nonetheless count the lionfish as one of the scarier creatures I have been called upon to treat.

Not all my unusual patients were in this category of "scary creatures"— tigers and elephants notwithstanding. Consider the domestic ferret (as distinct from the wild and rare black-footed ferret). Although many people cannot imagine having this close relative of the weasel and mink as a companion, in the 1980s and 90s particularly, the domestic ferret enjoyed a massive popularity boom. Pet shops could not keep up with the demand for young ferrets. Textbooks were written about the biology, medicine, and surgery of the domestic ferret, and seminars on ferret medicine and surgery became popular all over the country.

In spite of the fact that the domestic ferret was so popular and was an entirely different species from the wild ferret, the laws of some states, including Vermont, declared them to be a wild animal and thus illegal to keep as pets. The State Public Health Commissioner, Dr. Richard Vogt, declared war on the ferret, and he refused to acknowledge that the companion ferret was indeed a domesticated species and it had been so for hundreds and hundreds of years. He claimed they were dangerous and that they often attacked young children. It seemed to make no difference to him that veterinarians saw many more cat bites than occurred with ferrets. In fact, in all my practice time, I have never seen a case of a child bitten by a ferret. Because ferrets were classified as a wild species in our state, this meant that anyone wishing to own a ferret needed to get a permit from the Department of Fish and Wildlife. This was absurd, because ferrets were being sold quite openly in large numbers at almost every pet store in the greater Burlington area. What the regulation did do, however, was to make ferret owners reluctant to bring their pets to a veterinarian for medical care because they feared their "illegal" animals would be confiscated.

In spite of this fear, I saw quite a few ferret patients. Time and again, I argued with Dr. Vogt about the error of classifying the domestic ferret as a wild species simply because he did not feel they were an appropriate house pet. As for the argument that these ferrets could escape and become a troublesome wild species in Vermont, one had only to watch these creatures for a few minutes to appreciate the fact that they would much rather curl up in their bed, or in a lap, than hunt another animal. In fact, it would have been surprising if they even knew how to hunt, as they were quite content to eat the pellets of their commercial ferret chow.

The issue was finally resolved when the Vermont State Senate Agriculture Committee took up a bill stipulating that ferrets were, indeed, a domestic species and a legal animal to own. During the hearings preceding the vote, both Dr. Vogt and I were asked to testify on the question of whether domestic ferrets were, or were not, a wild creature that was potentially dangerous to humans. I would venture to say that any legislator who was present during my testimony would remember the occasion. I was so determined to see this absurd situation corrected that I brought one of my clients' ferrets to the hearing and plunked her down on the table in front of the committee members, challenging anyone to label this animal as a wild or dangerous creature. I think my case was pretty well made when the two-pound female curled up on the committee chairman's notepad and went to sleep. The bill passed with no difficulty.

Why would someone want a ferret as a pet? What caused them to be so wildly popular? Believe it or not, the fact is that ferrets have marvelous, mischievous, fun-loving personalities. An elderly couple who lived in a suburban neighborhood near Burlington owned two ferrets, named Fric and Frac because they always liked to get into playful, rough and tumble fracases. These ferrets were a delight to the couple, and they never tired of telling story after story about the tricks and situations of Fric and Frac.

For example, one early April afternoon the couple went grocery shopping, and when they returned they made several trips from the car to the house carrying in the bags of groceries. They put the groceries away, including some things that went into the refrigerator and the freezer compartment on the bottom level of their model of refrigerator. Fric and Frac, as always, greeted them at the door, as they often were fed treats after a grocery expedition. A few hours later, however, the couple noticed that Fric was missing. One of the challenging things about owning ferrets is keeping track of them, because they are superb tunnelers. Their shape and flexibility allows them to get into spaces that would be completely inaccessible to humans or most other animals. It wasn't too unusual for one or the other of this pair to disappear for awhile, but usually only for a relatively short time—Fric and Frac were pretty much inseparable.

By suppertime, Fric still hadn't appeared, and the couple began to search their house. When they didn't find him, they became convinced that he must have gotten outside while they were bringing in the groceries. They searched around their house, in their garden, and they searched their next door neighbors' properties—no Fric! But it was getting dark and they had to stop searching. They decided to resume the outside search next morning, and they searched the inside of their home once more. Fric still hadn't made an appearance, convincing them all the more that he was outside. Early April nights in Vermont are often very chilly, and the couple worried that Fric would be dangerously chilled; unlike their wild cousins, domestic ferrets do not have a thick hair coat.

Early the next morning the couple sat down to have a quick breakfast before searching the neighborhood again. One of them opened the bottom freezer door to get some orange juice concentrate and ... out crawled Fric! He had spent the night in freezing temperatures, all right—but not outside. He seemed fine and wanted to eat. But you can be sure that I received an early morning phone call telling me about Fric's freezer adventure and asking me to please make sure the little fellow was okay. Knowing how much these companions meant to this couple, I agreed to the early morning rendezvous. Fric passed his examination with flying colors, except that his tail had frostbite and he eventually lost the very tip. The couple was thrilled to have Fric back, and subsequently got a new refrigerator with the freezer compartment on the top, to insure this didn't happen again.

A second ferret story almost required the services of an MD, versus a DVM. A young couple, the McPhersons, likewise owned a pair of ferrets, whose very favorite game involved scampering up the stairs to the second floor of the home and launching themselves off the open balcony to land on the large, plush couch directly below. Where they learned to do this without first killing themselves is a tmystery, and frankly, I would not have believed it had the McPhersons not videotaped a sequence of the lively little creatures doing their trick three or four times in a row. It was quite a performance for any houseguest to watch, and the McPhersons were careful to warn anyone sitting on that couch that they could possibly get a sudden "visit" from above. Most of the McPhersons' friends and guests were young and free-spirited, so everyone got quite a charge out of the mischievous ferrets. However, one evening the McPhersons had an elderly aunt over for dinner, and because this relative was not particularly fond of animals, the couple had never told Auntie about the other members of their household. They had been very careful, they thought, to confine their two "performers" to an upstairs bedroom. After dinner, one of the McPhersons went upstairs to get something from the bedroom and ... you guessed it—the "Great Escape!" Eager to show their favorite trick to a new audience, the two acrobats launched themselves off the balcony and made perfect landings, one on each side of the tea-sipping guest.

I must rely here on Mr. McPherson's description of the ensuing excitement, but as he narrated it to me during the ferrets' next vaccination visit, the aunt let out a sound halfway between a scream and a squawk and turned so white that both Mr. and Mrs. McPherson were convinced she was having a heart attack. Mr. McPherson ran to call 911, while Mrs., not knowing what else to do, poured a healthy splash of brandy into a juice glass and administered it to the unprotesting, shocked aunt who, as it turned out, had not had an alcoholic beverage of any description for more than twenty years.

When the rescue squad arrived, their major task was to differentiate between a heart attack and intoxication!

With these stories of Princess, Anna Mae, Fric and Frac, and others, I have tried to convey the excitement and the challenge of treating some of my more unusual patients and their owners. As I relive these experiences, I marvel again and again at the scope of the education I received from my skilled and dedicated professors at the Ontario Veterinary College. In the following chapter, I will tell of my experiences with perhaps my most unique group of patients—about which even my professors, with all their wisdom and foresight, could not have anticipated the need for study.

chapter eleven

Reptiles and Their People

O f all the diverse creatures I have treated in my career, none has elicited such a complex mixture of fascination and fear as the reptiles—especially snakes. It would take a skilled psychologist to explain how both reactions very often occur in the same person, and as we will see, when treating reptile patients, most of the "treatment" must usually be directed to the owner. It is seldom a mysterious disease or condition of the reptile patient causing the problem; more often, it is the owner's lack of education on the husbandry and management of their reptile companion that results in a visit or call to the veterinarian.

Why do people choose to own reptiles? From a purely practical standpoint, reptiles do not bark or make noise, they do not require outdoor exercise, and many species do not require a large space. However, I believe it is the combination of fear and fascination that motivates both adults and children to purchase a snake, lizard, or turtle, and then face the challenge of creating a satisfactory environment as close to the natural habitat of the particular species as possible. This is often quite a costly undertaking, because reptile habitat is complicated. First, owners must provide a proper heat source, because reptiles do not have an internal mechanism to regulate their body temperature; they use their environment for temperature regulation. The habitat must also include a day/night light cycle with ultraviolet light; appropriate conditions of humidity or dryness, including a source of moisture, even for desert species; and suitable surroundings, including plantings, materials used in the bottom of the habitat, and items for shelter and concealment. Additionally, reptile owners must provide a proper diet according to the species requirements.

Where does a new reptile owner get accurate information and assistance to provide such an environment appropriate for the species selected? This critical information often comes from the pet store where the reptile is purchased. What is the training of the average pet store employee who sells such diverse species and advises the new owner? I have found great variation in the quality of the advice and the products sold by pet stores. Some genuinely seem to make an effort and some seem to be primarily interested in selling the products they carry, regardless of whether they are appropriate to the situation. It is to be hoped that the new owner has done some basic independent investigation before acquiring a reptile pet, but as we will see, this is often not the case.

My most challenging reptile patients have been turtles and tortoises. Imagine examining a turtle or tortoise, giving it medication, or even merely trimming its toenails. We all know what the natural reaction to those stressors will be—a retreat into the shell—and so the simplest procedure usually requires much innovation to accomplish. A surprising number of dedicated people keep these fascinating creatures as companion animals. With the possible exception of pond turtles, these reptiles are placid and surprisingly interactive with their owners. I have listened to story after story about how these unexpectedly intelligent animals have become part of a family for multiple generations.

The veterinarians who care for these beloved turtles and tortoises have had to develop techniques particularly suited to these armored creatures. For example, how might surgery be performed on a turtle? Why, by using a saw to remove a section of the bottom shell to expose the tissue underneath, and gluing or wiring it back in place after the surgery is completed, of course! Radiographs are routinely taken of turtles, and medications (usually by injection) are commonly given by the owner, whose dedication to his or her companion, for whatever the reason, seems often to exceed that of the owners of other reptile species.

Not all introductions to the owner of a particular reptile are direct; there is often an intermediary concerned third party. For example, one morning I took a call from a gentleman at the Vermont Department of Social Services. He requested an appointment for himself along with a father and son who were owners of a large red-tailed boa, which is one of the two most common snake species sold in this part of the country. These snakes are non-venomous and usually quite docile, but they are still completely wild creatures that must be respected as such at all times. The reason for this visit, the social services representative told me, was that the father was teaching his six-year-old son to carry their five-and-a-half-foot snake looped around his neck.

As the father explained to me, this was the "natural" position of the snake in the wild—looped around a tree branch to support its considerable body weight. I listened to the father's reasoning in utter amazement. Apparently, in his mind, there was no difference between his son's neck and a tree branch. The real heart of the problem, however, was that this man was absolutely convinced (as are many, many snake owners) that his snake was tame and would never act aggressively, especially with a member of the family. I tried to reason with the man, telling him of instance after instance where supposedly tame, regularly handled snakes had attacked their owners or handlers after years of non-aggressive behavior. I asked him why he was willing to risk his son's life if there was even a small chance of an accident.

But this owner was absolutely unshakeable. He knew his snake, he said. He'd taught his son the proper way to handle it so the snake would not feel threatened and therefore would not become aggressive. Never in the eight or nine years he had owned this snake had it shown the least sign of aggression. His final argument was that the only way his young boy could carry this large snake to show to his friends was to loop the snake around his neck and shoulders in this way!

I threw up my hands, turned to the gentleman from social services, who had been listening carefully to the entire dialogue, and said, "I've done my best, but I don't think I've been heard." Then I turned to the father and son, making sure the little boy was listening, and said very emphatically, "Make no mistake, sir, you are putting your son's life in danger." I felt, of course, like saying a good deal more to this obstinate, arrogant, foolish man, but I restrained myself.

As they left the hospital, the social services worker thanked me and said I would be hearing from him. And so I did, about one month later. The department had gone to court and had the snake confiscated from the father, who then was countersuing to regain possession of the boa. I could only hope that my words of warning might have sunk in. Alas, this was not my only worrying experience with snake owners.

Because Burlington, Vermont is a university town, one can find a generous supply of both students and bars. As I soon learned, college students and snakes apparently go together. But one combination that does not go together well is snakes and bars. I had received a call from a man who identified himself only as the owner of "a bar in the Burlington area." His problem was that a college student who frequented his bar had the annoying habit of bringing his pet python to the bar for an evening with the boys. The owner of the bar told him repeatedly not to bring the snake, but periodically this student either "forgot" or just stopped in for a quick one before going home.

Finally, the bar owner, who was reluctant to antagonize his student customers, had had enough of these antics and he determined to ask the local police to step in. Before he could do this however, the evening preceding the bar owner's call to me, the snake-owning student had lost his snake somewhere in the bar!

The bar owner was now faced with a dilemma. If he announced that there was a python loose in his bar and would the patrons please help look for it, he would probably lose most of his customers—permanently. If he kept the loss quiet and the snake suddenly made an appearance, he could potentially be faced with a customer so badly frightened that a lawsuit might result. Not to mention the code violations he was likely facing in either case. What he decided to do, he told me, was cross his fingers, say nothing about the wandering python, and announce that the bar would be closing early that evening for "inventory." After the last customer left, the owner locked the doors, and—although badly frightened by snakes—he and the student frantically searched every corner and cranny of the bar, but could not find the missing python. In desperation the next morning, he called me to find out how to lure the snake out into the open.

"What is the name of your establishment?" I asked.

"I'm sorry, but I can't tell you that. If word ever got out, I'd be ruined."

"Surely you understand that I need to see the physical set up of the bar in order to advise you how best to recapture this reptile," I told him. "Otherwise I don't know what the best way would be, other than to provide a warm spot in some corner and a small cage with some live mice in that same area."

He said, "Thank you," and immediately hung up.

For the next several days I carefully watched the local newspapers for any mention of a snake being captured or seen in a local bar, but to this day, I have no idea what actually happened—either to the snake, the student, or the bar.

Perhaps the most disturbing incident I had with snake owners was with a biology teacher at a regional high school. The teacher was an inspiring educator and had won many awards for his teaching excellence. I first came to know him by way of providing materials for some of his classroom demonstrations and by attending to his personal pets. However, it was more than two years later that I learned he was the owner of a large, very aggressive Burmese python, which he kept in his classroom in a homemade cage. The teacher himself was very wary of this snake (as well he should have been), so whenever it was necessary to handle the snake or clean the cage, he lowered the temperature in the room so the snake would become sluggish. Although this method increased safety, it was stressful for the snake's metabolism and certainly not the method an experienced reptile handler would use, even with an aggressive snake.

The way I learned about this classroom exhibit—this animal certainly could not be called a "pet"—was via one of the teacher's students, who brought the family dog to me for an annual checkup. I don't remember how we came to be discussing reptiles, but this student told me that he lived in mortal fear when he went into the biology classroom, because his seat was not far from the python's cage, and every time he (or any other student) got close to the cage, the snake would strike at the glass siding.

"What if the snake escaped?" he asked me. "Would it attack nearby people?"

Without having seen either the python or the classroom arrangement, I couldn't give a very good answer, but I did tell the fearful student that unless this snake were trapped or threatened, it was highly unlikely that anyone would be attacked. Alas, sure enough, during summer recess (when no students were in the classroom), the python did escape, and I got a call from the high school asking if I could help recapture it. The main concern—besides fear of the snake itself—was that the python would get into the ductwork of the heating system, which would make it almost impossible to retrieve. We were lucky enough to locate the python in the corner of a floor-level cupboard, and using two other helpers, I was able to restrain the animal safely and return it to the cage, after which we all breathed a great sigh of relief.

As diplomatically as I could manage, I suggested to the biology teacher that this animal was neither safe nor very instructive for his students, and that another reptile would be of far more educational value. But the python remained in the biology classroom for many more years. When faculty circumstances changed, it was impossible to find another home for the snake, and unfortunately, because of its aggressive nature, I was called upon to euthanize it.

These stories are meant to illustrate inappropriate management of wild creatures, which if in their native habitat would likely trouble no one. The stories are not meant to ridicule or to discourage anyone from interacting with these fascinating animals; however, it cannot be stressed enough that keeping these creatures in a captive situation does require significant commitment, effort, and forethought. But before I describe one of the most remarkable reptile-related episodes of my career, by way of contrast, I would like to tell a cautionary tale about the price of ignorance—there is just no other term for it. The difference, I believe, will be quite clear.

In the late summer of every year, the Champlain Valley Fair arrives in Essex Junction, Vermont—a weeklong exhibition of the area's agricultural heritage and industry, along with entertainment, carnival rides, and games. One year the carnival authorities decided to offer live baby green iguanas—tropical lizards—

as a prize for the ring-toss contest. This meant, of course, that anyone winning these iguanas gave no forethought about what was involved in caring for their "prize." Just step right up and win an iguana! Approximately three months after the fair, I entered my examination room at the Shelburne Veterinary Hospital to find a young lady, in her early 30s, holding two very small green iguanas. When she placed them on the examination table, I noted they were too weak to lift their heads off the mat. By this time in my career I had seen a lot of sick, debilitated animals, but very few were so weak as these two little lizards. Without much exception, and barring traumatic injury, most reptiles get sick slowly and they get better slowly because of their generally lower metabolic rates. It seemed these poor little creatures had been steadily getting weaker over a period of at least two or three weeks.

I admit that in the early days of my practice, my inclination would have been immediately to make a cross or scolding remark to this owner for letting things get to such a desperate state. But I swallowed hard, and prepared to take the history. My intentions were good; I wanted to help the young lady get these little ones better. Her first remark to me was, "I've only had them for three months, so I don't know much about them; I've just been feeding them iceberg lettuce."

I confess—something inside me snapped, and I said, "You've had these living creatures in your care for three whole months and you don't know much about them? When did you plan on learning?"

She began to cry, and I felt like a complete heel. I quickly apologized, but there was no way to get around the fact that these lizards were suffering from chronic malnutrition. Every bone in their bodies was visible and the bones were like rubber from lack of calcium and protein. For the next two days, I fed the lizards via tiny stomach tubes, bathed them in ultraviolet light (necessary for production of vitamin D3), warmed them to proper temperature, and gave them warm water soaks to correct their dehydration, but all to no avail. Both of them died within a half-day of each other—a very sad ending, made all the more so because it was 100 percent preventable.

The very next day, Dr. Fred Aliesky, whose practice was the closest to the Fairgrounds, and I went to see the executive director of the Champlain Valley Fair. Dr. Aliesky told the director of all the terribly sick kittens, puppies, and rabbits he saw every year after the Fair. I told the director the iguana story, and both of us made a strong plea for the fair to stop permitting vendors to offer live animals as prizes. Additionally, we implored that the director either stop allowing the sale of animals at the fair altogether, or at least require prior physical exams and more stringent housing regulations for those animals that were to be sold. It took more than a year of discussions, proposals, and counter-proposals, but finally, our requests were put into effect.

A much larger version of the "little lizard" problem came to my attention after a call I received on a Sunday afternoon from the veterinarian on emergency call. He had just received a call from a man who said he had a South American alligator that needed medical attention. I had, long before, given all the area veterinarians my home phone, and encouraged them to call me anytime they had questions or problems with birds, reptiles, or small mammals. So I returned the call from the alligator owner. Bear in mind that it was illegal to own this animal in the state of Vermont without a special permit. I identified myself and asked what the problem was.

"Do you know what a caiman is?" the man asked, rather belligerently.

"Yes," I answered. (A caiman is an incredibly adaptable crocodilian reptile found in Central and South America, and is in the same family as the American alligator.)

"Well, I've got one, and there's something in his eye."

Here was the cougar kitten situation all over again—a potentially unmanageable exotic species that did not belong in a private household. But there was no point in arguing with this man. The animal needed help, so I told him to bring the caiman in and I'd see what I could do. About an hour later a fellow in his early 20s came to the hospital with his caiman—a young one, twelve to fourteen inches in length. I immediately noticed a small piece of what looked like wood shaving in one eye.

"Okay," I said. "Just hold his mouth closed for a moment and I'll get that right out."

"No way; I'm not holding his mouth. He bites."

"But as you must know," I said, "the muscles that open his mouth are pretty weak, and especially at this age it will be easy to keep his mouth closed." (Anyone who has watched the numerous television programs on alligators or crocodiles knows about holding alligator jaws closed.)

"I'm not doing it. That's your job," said this owner.

In disgust, I made a simple gauze muzzle for the little fellow and tied his jaws closed. "Will you please at least hold his head still for a minute so I can get that shaving out of his eye. He can't hurt you."

Grudgingly, he held the head, and before he had a chance to change his mind, I quickly removed the foreign material from the eye using a tiny swab moistened with sterile saline.

"If you're afraid to handle him now when he's this size, what will you do when he gets bigger?" I asked. "And by the way, why did you get him in the first place?"

"I'll just turn him loose," said this incredible person. I couldn't believe what I was hearing.

"You mean you'll turn him loose here in Vermont? He surely won't survive in this climate."

"If I get back down to Florida, I'll release him there." This man was so unconcerned, so unaware of the implications of what he was saying, that I knew any discussion would be futile. Although veterinarians are not law-enforcement officials, I made up my mind that this man should be arrested and his "pet" caiman should be confiscated. As soon as he left the hospital, I called the nearest Department of Fish and Wildlife warden. Unfortunately, the caiman-owning scoundrel had given me a false name and address, knowing his reptile was illegal, and had paid me with cash. I hadn't thought to get his car license plate number. The Fish and Wildlife people were unable to track him down. As there were no reports of alligators in Lake Champlain—I am, of course, being facetious—I presume this caiman passed away, was brought elsewhere for any further care, or was released. Where the release might have occurred is anyone's guess.

As difficult as the above two episodes might be to understand, I have saved what I believe to be the most astounding story of reptilian ignorance and negligence for this next account, which involves a boy and his ... snake. It all began with what seemed to be a relatively routine first visit with a teenage boy and his mother, who brought in their just-purchased baby red-tail boa, which could not have been more than six inches in length.

As was usual for a first visit with a new reptile owner, I spent about a half-hour reviewing diet, temperature, and humidity requirements, habitat setup, and maintenance. Everything seemed to be going well until it came time to examine the little patient.

"If you'll just lift him out of his travel box, we'll go through the physical examination," I told the boy.

"I ain't touchin' him," was the reply.

I said, " I don't understand. Isn't this your snake? Didn't you just buy him?"

"Yeah, but I don't want to get bitten."

"Don't worry about that. Boas are usually quite easy to handle. Just move

Steven B. Metz, d.v.m.

slowly and handle him gently. Besides, this baby's teeth are so tiny you wouldn't even feel it even if he did bite." I felt it was important for the boy to handle the snake while in the office. Otherwise he might not feel confident about taking care of his snake at home.

"But what about the poison?" asked the boy.

I wasn't sure I had heard correctly. "What poison?"

"The snake is poisonous. That's why I don't want to handle him. That's why I brought him to you." I paused, incredulous. This boy actually thought he had a poisonous snake. And all the while, his mother was sitting in the exam room taking it all in, not saying a word. Presumably, then, she had agreed to her son bringing a poisonous snake into their home.

Trying to maintain some semblance of calm, I said, "Please listen carefully. Your snake is not poisonous. He is a boa constrictor, which means he gets his meals by wrapping around the food animal and squeezing tightly. No poison."

"What?" the boy shouted. "Not poisonous! We're taking him right back. Come on, Ma." And the two of them picked up the little box with the baby boa and marched out. I was so flabbergasted by the whole affair that I didn't even ask them to pay for the hour-long visit.

My last snake story is about one of my first and favorite reptile cases. It involved a high school student named Michael Cunningham who brought his young boa named Aaron (approximately fourteen inches in length) to see me, because Aaron had not eaten in several weeks. It is not unusual for snakes to stop eating for various reasons, especially during shedding or under conditions of lower temperatures or less sunlight. However, when I examined Aaron, I felt a firm lump about two-thirds of the way down his length through the underside of his body wall. Since this was a young snake, I didn't put a tumor very high on my list, but I was concerned about an intestinal blockage—possibly due to some poorly digested food material.

A radiograph showed some bones and other material in the intestine, and when I gave Aaron some barium via stomach tube—barium shows up bright white on x-ray as it travels down the length of the gastro-intestinal tract—the column of white could not get past this collection of bones and associated material. In other words, Aaron did, indeed, have an intestinal blockage, and that is why he wasn't eating.

The usual way to deal with an intestinal blockage in dogs and cats is to remove the blocking material surgically. But this type of surgery was not commonly performed on snakes. I certainly had never done it before now. I gave

Michael the option of taking Aaron down to Boston where there are surgeons with more experience, but this was impractical for the student. I explained to him that I had never done this particular surgery on a reptile before, but it didn't seem to worry him (as much as it worried me), and he urged me to operate and "fix" Aaron.

Hoping to get some helpful tips on reptile surgery, I picked up the phone and called the Franklin Park Zoo in the Boston area, because I was acquainted with the veterinarian there. When he came to the phone, I described my situation and asked what his success rate had been with snake intestinal surgery. To my great surprise, he said that he'd never done this surgery and didn't know anyone who had. We ended the conversation with him wishing me good luck. I was mostly on my own, but for moral support as well as the advantage of two minds considering the problem, I asked my good friend and colleague, Dr. Clint Reichard, to come and sit in on the surgery.

The first problem was the anesthesia. In a small snake, both heartbeat and respiration are slow and difficult to monitor. Deciding when Aaron was asleep enough to begin the surgery was tricky, and we took our time to be certain. The initial incision was quite different, too. Snakes and other reptiles have a large vein running along the centerline of their bellies, so the incision—through scales, not skin—had to be off the centerline, which is different from most mammalian abdominal surgery.

Once inside the coelom (like birds, reptiles do not have separate chest and abdominal compartments), I found the distended, discolored section of intestine that was blocked. As in the case of the Doberman puppy that had swallowed a pair of stockings a few years earlier, I was hoping the involved intestine was still healthy so I would not have to perform a resection and anastomosis—in other words, remove the damaged intestinal segment and rejoin the two healthy ends.

The wall of the little snake's intestine seemed to be paper-thin, so I made a very gentle incision, as small as possible, and removed the bones and hair of Aaron's last mouse meal. I then selected some tiny suture material and carefully stitched up the intestinal incision. The sutures seemed to hold securely, so I prepared to close the primary coelomic incision.

"What's that?" my colleague asked suddenly, pointing to a dark-colored structure just forward of the section of intestine I'd just sutured together. If the situation hadn't been quite as tense, I would have burst out laughing. If Doc Reichard wanted a lesson in reptile anatomy, he'd surely come to the wrong establishment. So I half-growled at him, "How the hell do I know? This is my first time." He gave me a big grin, and said, "Let's have all this down by next time, professor." The rest of the surgery went smoothly and Aaron's recovery proceeded uneventfully. When he finally ate his next yummy mouse, we all cheered.

Seven years later, in 1984, I took a phone call: "Dr. Metz, it's Michael Cunningham, owner of Aaron, the boa constrictor you operated on a few years ago."

"Of course, Michael. I certainly haven't operated on that many snakes since Aaron's little problem. How can I help you?"

"Aaron seems to have gotten himself into a little trouble, starting a few days ago."

"Uh oh, what is it this time?" I asked with a sinking feeling.

"My roommate took the strings off of his guitar, and Aaron crawled in. Now he won't come out."

I was trying to picture this, and the first question I asked was, "Can't you simply pull Aaron out of the guitar?"

"I'm afraid not," Michael explained. "You see, Aaron has grown quite a bit since you last saw him. He's about five feet long now, and very strong. He just won't budge. This is a pretty valuable guitar, Dr. Metz. Can you help us?"

I thought for a moment, and then said, "Yes, I think I can help you get Aaron out of the guitar. Why don't you bring him, er, I mean the guitar down to the hospital in about an hour. It might be a good idea to have your roommate bring the guitar strings down, too, so we can prevent this from happening again."

Two hours later, Michael, his roommate, the guitar (quite a bit heavier with the addition of Aaron), and a reporter from the Burlington Free Press newspaper gathered in the larger of my two examination rooms. My plan was actually quite simple, although depended somewhat on Aaron being reasonably good-natured about giving up his cozy abode. I would pipe anesthetic vapor into the guitar until Aaron relaxed enough to allow removal. One possible complication—and I made sure to discuss this with Michael before I began—was that since I couldn't see Aaron, it would be hard to judge the amount of anesthesia needed to relax him enough. So I took things very gradually, much more gradually than I would have if I had the patient out in front of me to assess depth of relaxation. Periodically, I had Michael reach into the guitar and "test" Aaron's muscle strength.

After thirty minutes of gradual increase in the concentration of anesthetic in the guitar, Michael reached in and was able to start removing length after length of reluctant boa from the guitar. By the time Aaron made his grand exit, we were astonished that so much snake could fit into such a small space. All this time, the Free Press reporter was snapping pictures, and when the story came out in next day's newspaper with the headline "Boa Frets Great Guitar Escape," the pictures showed some pretty interesting facial expressions on all the onlookers as Aaron was reeled out of the guitar. The story was so novel that it was picked up by USA Today and the Boston Globe, and for many months I heard plenty of jokes about interfering with the area's latest musical talent and frightening my patients so badly that they hid in unsuspected places. But all's well that ends well, and Michael Cunningham (and Aaron) went on to graduate from the University of Vermont College of Medicine. I thought surely my relationship with Aaron was over, as I understood that Michael was moving out of state.

About twenty years later, our youngest son, Jamie, was about to graduate from the University of Vermont College of Medicine, and had decided he wanted to be a pediatrician. In choosing a residency where he could take his specialty training, he settled on Seattle Children's Hospital as one of the most outstanding programs in the country. In the spring of 2006, Jamie flew out to Seattle for a series of interviews at the hospital. As he walked down the halls of Seattle Children's Hospital, he was wearing a doctor's white coat that had "University of Vermont" stenciled on it. Suddenly, he felt a tap on his shoulder, and a gentleman passing by in the hall said to him, "Are you from Vermont?" Jamie admitted to being from Vermont.

Next question: "Where in Vermont are you from?"

"The greater Burlington area," Jamie told him.

"Do you happen to know a veterinarian by the name of Dr. Steven Metz?"

Not sure where this was leading, Jamie cautiously replied, "He's my father."

The gentleman then said, "Please tell him Michael Cunningham and Aaron say hello."

It turned out that Michael was a pediatrician in the Seattle area and had become quite well known as the medical director of the Cranio-Facial Center and division chief of Cranio-Facial Medicine at Seattle Childrens' Hospital. That evening we got a call from Jamie, who asked me if I remembered a Michael Cunningham.

"Of course," I said. "He's the medical student whose snake I removed from a guitar twenty years ago."

"Who's Aaron—his son?" asked Jamie.

"No, his boa."

We all had a good laugh over the amazing coincidence, and Dr. Cunningham and Aaron may well have put in a "good word" for Jamie, who was accepted into the highly competitive Pediatric Residency program. In fact, Dr. Cunningham became Jamie's advisor throughout his training, and when Connie and I traveled to Seattle for a visit with Jamie, it was quite a thrill for me to meet this distinguished M.D. whom I'd known since he was in high school. Unfortunately, Aaron passed away shortly after our visit, but he remains one of the most fondly remembered patients of my career.

chapter twelve

It's the People

I have often been accused of paying more attention to my patients than to my clients—the owners. I cannot deny that many times I have had to get up off the floor of my examination room where I've been "communicating" with an especially appealing puppy, kitten, or adult dog or cat, and I've had to remind myself to greet the owner and introduce myself. In spite of this bias, to which I freely admit, in forty-one years of practice there have been many clients who have enriched my life and career, taught me great lessons, and who have frequently prompted serious soul-searching about what is truly important in life. To avoid embarrassing anyone who has challenged or inspired me as a veterinary practitioner, I have changed the names of some of these memorable clients.

Around Christmastime every year, companion animal veterinarians brace themselves for cases where pets have eaten any (or all) of the following: the tinfoil that covered the turkey, Christmas tree ornaments, ribbon or string, jewelry, holly berries, chocolate, insulated fireplace gloves, and many other such enticing morsels. These are all items that I have had to remove, one way or another, from dog, cat, ferret, or bird digestive tracts (reptiles seem either to be more discriminating or more tolerant of strange material). However, once in a while, even the most experienced veterinary practitioner can be surprised by pet gastronomic adventures.

One year, a week before Christmas, I was not initially surprised to find Mrs. Hamilton and her grey miniature poodle, Rosie, in my examination room. There are owners from whom it is difficult to obtain a history and information about the reason for a visit; this was not the case with Mrs. Hamilton, however. This is what I learned within sixty seconds of her entrance into the examination room: Mrs. Hamilton's guest list for the week (along with some juicy tidbits of gossip about each guest); her family's plans for the New Year's holiday; the dinner menu for the week; summaries of interesting articles she had recently read in newspapers and magazines, and also, by the way, Rosie had eaten a small, metallic Christmas tree ornament. The ornament was of great sentimental significance and I was informed of its history from the day it was manufactured. I often felt that I should have supplemental oxygen ready during a visit from Mrs. Hamilton, because, somehow, she was able to tell me all this without stopping to take a breath. I also wished for an experienced court reporter to take down what she said, because all of her information was delivered at machine-gun pace.

When I finally was able to slow Mrs. Hamilton down long enough to get a few pertinent details about Rosie's indiscretion—such as when she had swallowed the ornament, whether she eaten since the accident, and what, if anything, was being produced at the other end of her digestive tract—I suggested we x-ray Rosie's abdomen to locate the ornament. Mrs. Hamilton readily agreed, while describing for me her own last personal x-ray experience.

Rosie was a very cooperative patient, and the abdominal films showed that the small piece of metal had passed through the stomach and into the first part of the small intestine. Because she was eating well and acting normally, I felt chances were very good that she would pass the ornament without difficulty. I suggested to Mrs. Hamilton that she use a stick to "dissect" what Rosie passed and look for the ornament over the next two or three days. Mrs. Hamilton agreed to do so, although she was a bit concerned that her neighbors would think the activity strange, and she made sure to describe each of her neighbors' family situations.

On the second day after the initial visit, I took a deep breath and called Mrs. Hamilton to find out if Rosie had passed the metallic ornament. She was very glad to hear from me and gave me an hour-by-hour account of her efforts to locate the Christmas tree ornament in Rosie's "poops" (her preferred terminology). She reported that so far, she had been unable to find it. To allay her fears that the ornament would become stuck, I had her bring Rosie in for a follow-up abdominal film, which showed the metallic piece near the end of the digestive tract. Sure enough, the next day I received a triumphant call from Mrs. Hamilton describing in great detail just how she found the ornament, and discussed her dilemma of whether or not to clean and use the ornament on her tree—in light of what it had "been through."

I was very happy that Rosie had not needed surgery to resolve this problem because I felt that had this been the case I would have been the one needing supplemental oxygen. I sincerely hoped that the rest of the holiday season would pass uneventfully for Mrs. Hamilton and Rosie. However, this was not to be, for the day before Christmas Mrs. Hamilton called to report that Rosie had eaten some delicious Lake Champlain Chocolates. She not only was able to tell me exactly how many Rosie had eaten, but also what flavor she had seemed to prefer—caramel. Mrs. Hamilton wasn't sure exactly why chocolate was dangerous for dogs, but she reviewed two articles for me that she had read listing chocolate as a potential cause of canine death.

In fact, Mrs. Hamilton was quite correct. Chocolate contains, among other substances, theobromine. When consumed by dogs, theobromine can act like an overdose of caffeine, causing dangerous increases in blood pressure and heart rate, all of which can be fatal. Using the National Animal Poison Control Center calculations, I was able to determine that Rosie had not eaten a lethal amount of chocolate, and once again, she was eating her own food and acting normal. There is no specific reversal agent for chocolate overdose, so I advised Mrs. Hamilton to be alert for Rosie showing clinical signs of panting, shaking, restlessness, or personality change, and to call immediately if any of these signs occurred.

Christmas and the following days passed without event. But the day before New Year a familiar voice on the phone told me, "Dr. Metz, Rosie is acting like she has a needle in her rear end." Mrs. Hamilton then described all the signs of discomfort that Rosie had been exhibiting for the past twelve to fourteen hours. Resignedly, I said, "Bring her right in, Mrs. Hamilton."

Rosie came trotting in just a few minutes later looking as if nothing ever happened to her. I examined, I poked, and I prodded— no reaction. By this time, I was convinced that Mrs. Hamilton felt that Rosie ought to have at least a weekly checkup, so I decided to humor this highly excitable owner. I put on a latex exam glove and gently inserted my finger into Rosie's rectum. Immediately, I froze in that position and asked Mrs. Hamilton incredulously, "How in heaven's name did you know?" Wedged exactly crosswise in Rosie's rectum was, in fact, a sewing needle.

I gave Rosie a light anesthetic, reached in with a wire-cutting scissors, cut the needle in half, and removed the pieces. Mrs. Hamilton examined the needle and said, "Yes, that's the one I've been missing." She reached into her large purse, pulled out an elegantly monogrammed linen napkin she had been mending, and proceeded to describe exactly why she had to use that particular type of needle for that particular type of stitch.

As incredible as it may seem, Rosie had apparently swallowed the needle, which had then made its way through the entire length of the gastrointestinal tract and had only gotten stuck at the far end. Through all of these adventures, Rosie's grey whiskery face never changed expression, and she was obviously much calmer about things than we humans were.

That same year, I attended my very first cat show, held annually in Burlington at the Sheraton Hotel Conference Center. I had been to many dog shows, even competing with my own dogs, but as I quickly found out, a cat show is a completely new world. I went to this cat show because of one specific cat in my practice whose name was Garage. Shortly before this cat show, Garage's owner—a very nice, laid-back young lady—brought him in for a checkup and a health certificate. Health certificates are usually required for travel, so I asked her if she and Garage were taking a trip. No, she replied. She was going to enter Garage in the cat show. She felt he had a great chance to win the show's award for "Best Personality". I soon learned that at a cat show, in addition to the competition within the recognized breeds, there were all sorts of other prizes awarded: a prize for the fluffiest tail, for the bluest eyes, for the most striking markings, and for the best personality of all the cats in the show.

It was enough of a surprise to find out about all these "special awards," but that Garage should be entered for this particular prize was more surprising because every time Garage came to see me he exhibited the personality of a man-eating shark. I could hear his cat-swearing (cat owners will understand this descriptive reference) from the moment he entered the hospital reception area, and in the examination room, I counted myself fortunate if Garage tolerated my attempts to examine his eyes and ears with a light source held a respectful distance from his face.

Listening to his heart and lungs was out of the question. All that could be heard was amplified growling, for which I certainly didn't need a stethoscope. Feeling his abdomen or examining his skin was almost guaranteed to earn me a lightning-fast slap from a front paw. Any attempt to check his mouth or teeth was tantamount to asking for a trip to the hospital emergency room. Garage's owner always insisted that my veterinary hospital was the only place Garage acted this way. At home, he was "a lamb," a perfect gentleman, and she wanted to prove it by entering him in the personality competition. "Why don't you come and watch?" asked Garage's owner.

So that is how I found myself standing in the audience gathered around the stage where the cat personality judging was to take place. There were small portable cages holding four or five other cats—a fluffy Persian, a sleek Siamese, a Scottish fold, and a Maine coon cat—and there was Garage, whose lineage was far less distinguished, although that did not matter for this particular award.

The judging procedure itself was great entertainment. The judge wore glasses with whiskers attached to the outside edges, and she produced an astonishing collection of sounds that apparently were meant to interest the competitors on the stage. Her procedure for assessing the personality of each cat was to reach into the cage, lift him or her out, and with one hand raise the cat high over her head. Apparently, if the cat had the "best personality," this position would be enjoyable and the cat would be completely relaxed. Lowering the cat to chest level, the judge then flipped each contestant on her side and on her back, stood the cat on her front paws and on her hind paws—all of which was supposed to be completely agreeable and enjoyable to the "best personality" contender. The final test was to see if the judge could get the cat to play with a tempting toy, and never have I seen such a collection of cat toys as that judge had piled on the stage.

During the judging, I tried to observe the condition of the arms and hands of this judge to see how badly she had been wounded while performing her manipulations and assessments. Although I didn't see any bandages, I did note that Garage seemed to be the last kitty on her schedule. As she approached his cage, I stepped back apprehensively and scanned the area for a first aid station; I was certain this judge would need one very shortly. I also waited for the growling, hissing, and swearing demonstration in which my experience had ascertained that Garage was certainly proficient.

To my amazement, Garage went completely limp and started purring loudly the minute the judge opened the cage door. She plucked him out of the cage, twisted him upside down, right side up, and sideways—he never stopped purring. He played with all the toys, he rolled over on his back, and as a final demonstration of his outstanding personality, he allowed the judge to drape him around her neck like a fur collar. I felt a tap on my shoulder. "Now do you believe me?" asked his owner, who had been watching my reaction as much as her cat's. As I turned to answer, I heard the judge announce the winner of the "Best Personality in the Show"—none other than good old Garage!

I was convinced. I decided that the next time Garage came to my hospital for a checkup, I would act just like the judge at the cat show (minus the whiskery glasses— I could not find a similar pair). When the day arrived to try my new Garage-charming technique, I tried to imitate some of the sounds the judge had made, and without hesitation—ignoring the growls and cat swear words—I unlatched the door to Garage's carrier. I never got the chance to reach into the carrier for out from the carrier door came a left jab that would have done credit to Muhammad Ali—and I was the recipient of five parallel scratches on the back of my hand. It was a good reminder to never suspend my own judgment about a patient—no matter who had "judged" him in the past.

The second or third year after I started my practice at the Shelburne Veterinary Hospital, a petite elderly lady came through the front door with a huge male bloodhound on the end of her leash—or perhaps, I thought, it was she who was at the end of the leash and the bloodhound was taking her into the hospital. When most people think of the bloodhound dog breed, they think of a wonderful, friendly dog with lots of wrinkles, big jowls, and a waggly tail that always finds the lost child or tracks an escaped criminal, then licks him to death. When I think of bloodhounds, I think of Joe and his owner, the petite Dr. Charlotte Woodruff.

At this stage of my growing practice, I was very happy to welcome any new client, and usually I quickly got down on the floor and introduced myself to the new patient. But there was a very obvious low rumble coming from my new patient and I couldn't see his eyes because of all his wrinkles. I am often asked, "How often do you get bitten, Doctor, while you're handling strange dogs, poking lights in their ears and at their eyes, putting your hands in their mouths, and doing many other things they don't like?"

In my case the answer to this question is that I have been bitten only once in my career. It is true, however, that during the course of a thorough physical examination, we veterinarians do things that are not popular with our patients. The veterinary practitioner who wishes to keep all of his or her fingers, eyes, ears, and other vital appendages, must develop the skill of reading their patients' expressions, and they must do it within the first few seconds of entering the examination room. If their assessment is incorrect, they are at risk of injury, sometimes life-threatening or career-ending injury. There is a definite art to reading the attitude of an animal—usually expressed by such things as body posture, type of movement, and vocalization. This is true throughout the animal kingdom, from insects and fish to humans. It is up to the veterinarian to become skilled in recognizing these signs and to handle the patient accordingly. It is also up to the veterinarian, as we have seen in the previous episode with Garage, not to suspend his or her own judgment on the word of an owner.

Back to Dr. Woodruff and Joe, the bloodhound. Not being able to see Joe's eyes, I couldn't accurately assess Joe's intentions. All other signs told me that Joe was saying, "Don't mess with me." Throughout my career, I have firmly believed in listening to what my patient is telling me, in addition to what the owner says. In Joe's case, this proved to be a fortunate decision, because when I asked Dr. Woodruff what the purpose of today's visit was, she said, "This is a get-acquainted visit. Joe didn't get along very well with his previous veterinar-ian." With some reluctance, I got Dr. Woodruff to tell me who that practitioner was. Dr. Woodruff insisted it was the veterinarian's own fault that he and Joe didn't get along; he had not approached Joe "the right way." As far as the growl-ing that Joe was now producing, Dr. Woodruff said, "Oh don't pay any attention to that. He's just talking." He certainly is, I thought to myself, and I'll bet I know exactly what he's saying.

I had recently purchased an Elsam restraint table—a hydraulically operated examination table. A very knowledgeable veterinary practitioner designed this marvelous piece of equipment for two purposes: to save the backs of veteri-narians and their technicians, who otherwise would have to lift patients up to the standard examination table, and to restrain an aggressive or unruly patient without danger to either the veterinarian or the patient. This eliminated the need for a technician to restrain the patient physically. Some practitioners don't care for this equipment, but many times this table allowed me to work safely with animals that would have either required sedation or would have posed a risk to my staff or me. Joe the bloodhound was a perfect candidate for the Elsam table—he weighed 128 pounds and, despite Dr. Woodruff's assertions, in my judgment he was a scary and dangerous animal.

During my initial examination of Joe, I learned that Dr. Woodruff, herself, was actually afraid of him. When I went to examine his ears, she warned me that he didn't care to have them touched, even by her. This was unfortunate be-cause Joe had yeast infections in both ears. Thanks to the restraint table, I was able to examine and treat the ear infection—the first time this had been done, said Dr. Woodruff, in a long time.

My judgment about Joe was vindicated the next day when I spoke with his previous veterinarian. It seems that Joe resented something the doctor did and so he knocked the veterinarian to the floor and tried to rip his throat apart! Dr. Woodruff weighed about 110 pounds, lost most of her sight in one eye, and was somewhat frail. Joe outweighed her by almost twenty pounds and was a very powerful canine. In my opinion, here was a clear case of an inappropriate animal for this owner. But Dr. Woodruff and her now deceased husband had owned bloodhounds for years, and I was (in her opinion) definitely not knowl-edgeable enough about the breed to advise her on such matters. So be it! If Dr. Woodruff insisted on keeping Joe, I knew it was my obligation to keep him as healthy and problem-free as possible. When Joe passed away a few years and many harrowing visits later, Dr. Woodruff went right out and adopted a large, male bluetick hound that, although not nearly as aggressive as Joe had been, was every bit as resistant to veterinary attention. Sometimes we veterinarians just can't win.

In the greater Burlington area there is the Champlain Valley Kennel Club, a group of dog breeders and owners who compete with their dogs in conformation and obedience shows and trials. The Club hosts a large dog show every year in July at the Essex Fair Grounds, and as the weather at that time of the year is apt to be quite hot and humid, the Club was concerned about heat stroke, and rightfully so. Dogs and cats are very susceptible to heat stroke, because unlike horses or humans, they do not have sweat glands in their skin. The primary way they cool themselves is by panting—that is, air exchange. So if, for example, a dog is kept in a car in the sun, even with the windows open, the temperature in the car will soon rise to well over 106-110 degrees. A dog's normal body temperature ranges from 100-102.4 degrees. Therefore, in this example, when the dog is panting it is breathing out air of 102 degrees and taking in air of 106 degrees or higher. The outcome is easily predictable.

In the interest of furthering the education of its members, the Kennel Club invited veterinarians from around the area to speak on different topics of concern. I happened to be the attending veterinarian for one year's upcoming dog show and I was invited to give a lecture just before the show on prevention and treatment of heat stroke. In this lecture, I made sure to mention that when heat stroke is suspected the dog's temperature must be taken to verify the diagnosis. I also emphasized that it was not adequate to simply wet the patient down with cold water; there needed to be a deep tub with ice so a dog suffering from heat stroke could be completely surrounded with cooling liquid. During the talk I noticed several club members taking careful notes, particularly Mrs. Nonie Cordner, an extremely energetic, experienced golden retriever breeder, and an officer in the club. I particularly enjoyed talking to this group because they asked many very intelligent and thought-provoking questions, from a viewpoint quite different from that of a gathering of veterinarians.

As feared, the weather on the day of the dog show was very hot and humid. The judging rings were under a tent that provided shade, and most competitors found areas on the fairgrounds that were shaded or they had air-conditioned vehicles, some of which were quite luxurious campers or trailers. As it turned out, the air-conditioning turned out to be a mixed blessing, because when a dog kept in a heavily air-conditioned vehicle stepped outside, the sudden change in temperature was not always tolerated very well. This is exactly what happened to a large male Bernese mountain dog with a heavy black-hair coat; he stepped out of his air-conditioned camper into the heat, walked part way to the show ring and collapsed.

Like a well-trained emergency medical team, Kennel Club members quickly converged on this 135-pound dog and carried him to the show supervisor area where a water hose had been connected. Within a matter of seconds, long-time club member and my great friend, Joanne Martin, had a thermometer in the dog, and as I answered the page and came to the supervisor area Nonie Cordner was dragging a large galvanized metal tub filled half-way up with ice. Joanne reported that the dog's temperature was over 106 (off the end of the thermometer scale), and we all lifted the dog into the tub of ice and began filling it with water.

Recent studies on the effects of heat stroke had shown that proper treatment involves more than just cooling the patient down. The high body temperature can cause severe organ damage; therefore, intravenous corticosteroids should be given as quickly as possible. There was a slight problem doing that in this case, however, because most of the dog was in the ice bath. My underwater intravenous injection to this soggy Bernese mountain dog is surely a candidate for the most acrobatic venipuncture of my career. I had to climb into the ice bath with the dog to give the injection, but I'm happy to report that both the heat-stroke victim and the iced veterinarian recovered fully. If the alert and attentive members of the Champlain Valley Kennel Club had not had the deep tub full of ice readily available, it might well have been a different story.

Other examples of owners who listened carefully to veterinary advice include a young animal-loving couple, George and Elizabeth Goodrich, who owned a flock of sheep, several horses, and four large dogs. The dogs were well taken care of, but because they were able to roam freely on the Goodriches' property, they frequently had adventurous encounters with the resident wildlife. Consequently, I was well used to responding to calls at all hours of the day and night. But nothing could have prepared me for the day the Goodriches transformed the Shelburne Veterinary Hospital into a M*A*S*H* unit.

It had been a relatively quiet morning and we were just finishing the surgical schedule for the day. I had one technician and a receptionist in the hospital. We were preparing to take a break for lunch when the front door burst open and George Goodrich came in carrying one of his dogs, closely followed by Elizabeth with the other three dogs on leashes.

For a moment I didn't quite recognize the dogs. There was something different about them. They all looked as if their faces had been dipped in cream or vanilla frosting. When I got closer, I realized the white color was due to a solid mass of porcupine quills. I couldn't see any trace of skin between the quills. Each dog must have egged on the others to continue attacking the porcupine. In all my years of practice, I have never seen such terrible cases of quilling. There were quills in the nostrils, around the eyes, inside the mouth, and two of the dogs had quills in their front paws. I thought to myself, this porcupine must be bald. It couldn't possibly have any quills left!

I had always emphasized to my clients that it is important to remove quills as quickly as possible because the quills become softer as time passes and they will often become more deeply embedded—which makes removing them more difficult. There have been cases in which quills have perforated or lodged in internal organs. The Goodriches had listened carefully to that advice, and when "their turn" came, they didn't hesitate to bring the dogs to the hospital.

I had examined these dogs recently and knew them all to be in good physical condition, and so I administered a light general anesthesia to the four of them, one after another. Then I set my technician and my receptionist to removing quills from the first two dogs, while I instructed George and Elizabeth in the "art" of pulling out quills without breaking them off. Then I started them in a quill-removal assembly line. I was the roving quill removal supervisor and anesthetist. When any of the dogs showed signs of awakening from their anesthesia, I administered additional medication as needed, and when there was a quill in a particularly difficult area, such as close to an eye, or in the back of the throat, I performed the removal.

For the next hour and a half to two hours, I felt as if I were on roller skates. There were anesthetized dogs in my treatment room and in both my examination rooms; there were bowls and bowls full of quills all over the hospital. It was a truly gruesome scene. But all's well that ends well—the four dogs recovered quickly with no side effects. I give the Goodriches full credit for heeding my advice about treating porcupine incidents immediately; it likely made all the difference in the healing time for their dogs.

What happens, though, when a client asks for the advice of a veterinary practitioner, then disregards it?

In 1997, the City Council of Burlington asked me, along with the city's Animal Control Officer, to address some concerns about the spread of rabies in the greater Burlington area. This came about because after many years without rabies in Vermont, the early 1990s saw fox rabies came down from Canada as part of a twenty-year cycle we seem to experience. At the same time, some

S T E V E N   B .   M E T Z ,   D . V . M .

"sportsmen" brought a number of raccoons up to our region from southern states in order to have animals for their coonhounds to hunt. Unfortunately, some of these transplanted raccoons were infected with rabies. The rabid animals subsequently infected the local population of skunks and raccoons. The infection spread rapidly, and by 1994, raccoon rabies, which affects most other mammals as well, was firmly established in Vermont. After two cases of rabies were reported in the city of Burlington, the City Council decided to discuss ways to increase the safety of its residents.

The Animal Control Officer and I suggested that there were some obvious precautions that could be taken, such as placing garbage in raccoon-proof containers, avoiding outdoor feeding of cats and dogs, and a more strict enforcement of dog licensing. Then I addressed a "sacred" subject—free-roaming cats. I cited a study that showed that outdoor cats were much more likely to be exposed to rabies-carrying wildlife than were dogs; there were three times as many cases of rabies in domestic outdoor cats as there were in dogs. Studies also showed clearly that owners of free-roaming cats were less likely to get their cats vaccinated against rabies. I proposed that the City of Burlington enact a cat-licensing ordinance, similar to dog licensing. This would encourage owners to keep their cats from roaming the city streets and neighborhoods, help to identify any cat involved in a biting incident, and most importantly—because any animal to be licensed had to have a certificate of vaccination against rabies—this ordinance would increase the number of vaccinated cats. People come in contact with domestic animals much more frequently than wildlife, so the more domestic animals that get vaccinated against rabies, the better the barrier between the rabies virus and people.

I further proposed that the city take a census of homeowners and tenants in order to know, as accurately as possible, how many dogs and cats lived in Burlington. This would be a good summer project for high school or college students, and the cost would be more than offset by the fees collected from the increased number of dog, and now cat, licenses issued.

From the reaction these two proposals provoked, however, one would have thought I had suggested that the city of Burlington secede from the state of Vermont! It seemed unimaginable to the Council members that cat owners could be persuaded to keep their cats indoors, despite the many health concerns caused by free-roaming cats, to say nothing of the high probability of these cats getting hit by cars, chased or attacked by dogs, or getting into fights with other free-roaming cats (whose rabies vaccination status was, of course, unknown).

After about a half hour of heated discussion, one Council member stood up and said, "Why are we wasting time on this? We have very important matters to discuss; we have potholes in many of our streets that need attention."

I watched in amazement as they tabled the rabies discussion indefinitely. Hadn't they asked me to come to the meeting with information and to make recommendations? Even after a Burlington police officer was chased down the sidewalk on the north side of the city by a rabid skunk, the Burlington City Council never again, to my knowledge, discussed the matter of licensing cats or taking a pet census.

Another story of veterinary advice going unheeded involves a pleasant young man named Dan who brought his male German shorthair pointer puppy to the hospital for a routine examination and vaccination visit. This was the breed of dog that had been members of my family since 1965, so I made a big fuss over this puppy and told many stories about Kin, my first German short-hair, as well as some observations and recommendations on living a happy life with this breed. In handling the puppy, I got the impression that he was a little standoffish, and I advised Dan, who hoped to use him for bird hunting, to make sure to socialize the young dog very well. By this time in my experience I had owned five German shorthairs, had handled and treated many more, and it was very rare to have an aggressive shorthair, but certainly some were more outgoing than others.

Several weeks later, the puppy, now almost six months of age, came in for his final vaccinations. This is the age at which male dogs are commonly neutered (although it can be done at almost any age after three to four months). During this visit, I learned that there was a "little problem" with the pup. He was growling at Dan's wife—never at Dan. It was a problem of dominance, Dan thought, and he was encouraging his wife to be firm with the puppy.

I listened to this with considerable concern. It is not very common for a dog at this young age to exhibit obvious aggressive behavior, and when it did happen, the behavior was almost certain to become more pronounced as the dog grew older. I advised Dan to have the pup neutered as soon as possible and to take him to a board-certified behavior specialist. There was only one such specialist in Vermont—luckily not too far away.

Unfortunately, Dan didn't act on either of my recommendations. He didn't neuter his dog because he thought it would spoil him for hunting, and he didn't consult with a behavior specialist. What he did do was get on the Internet, where he found someone who claimed to be a behavior expert—I never found

S t e v e n   B.   M e t z ,   D . V . M .

out what credentials this person claimed to have—and this "expert" gave Dan's wife the following advice. She needed to establish that she was the alpha person in the family pack. Therefore, she should grab the dog's cheeks, stare directly into his eyes, then roll him over on his back and hold him down. Can anyone predict what happened when Dan's wife attempted these maneuvers? The next call I received from Dan was from the Medical Center emergency room, where they were stitching up his wife's face. He called to tell me that he had arranged for a friend to take the dog to the nearest veterinary hospital and have him put to sleep. What a tragic and likely unnecessary ending!

A final case of ignored veterinary advice involves raccoons. I have mentioned that rabies, especially in raccoons, came to Vermont in the early 1990s. There were frequent stories about rabies and raccoons on local radio stations and in the newspapers. In spite of all the publicity, some owners (even affluent, well educated ones) still neglected to have their pets, especially their cats, vaccinated properly, and some people still thought raccoons were cute and continued to feed them on their porches. For sheer dangerous and—dare I say—irresponsible behavior, nothing matches the series of phone calls I received from a single mother with two young children.

In the first call from the mother—I never learned her name—she asked me if there were vaccinations for baby raccoons. I told her that no vaccine had been approved for raccoons because they were, of course, wildlife. This young mother then told me that she had adopted a baby raccoon that seemed to be an orphan. She had taken the little creature into her house; her two children adored the baby and they were helping her take care of it. She asked what medical care was needed for pet raccoons. For the second time during that phone call, I emphasized that raccoons should not be kept as pets and that they were a potential danger, health wise, to her children and herself. There were specially trained and licensed rehabilitators for orphaned or injured wildlife, I told her, and if she would bring the baby raccoon down to my hospital, I would see that the little one was properly taken care of.

No, she said, the raccoon seemed to be doing well in her home; it looked perfectly healthy, was eating well, her children loved it and she wanted to keep it. She was afraid that if she brought the baby raccoon down to my hospital, I would either put it to sleep myself, or turn it over to a Vermont Fish and Wildlife warden who would put it to sleep. I asked her name and where she was calling from so I could get a rehabilitator to call her, but she hung up the phone.

About ten days later, I received a second call from this unidentified woman.

This time she was a little concerned. It seemed that the baby raccoon was doing a lot of sneezing, there was a discharge coming from the nose and eyes, and its appetite was decreased.

"Can you give me some medication or tell me what to do for him?" she asked.

"I just can't," I said. "I'd have to know what's wrong with him and how much he weighs. Veterinary dosages depend on body weight, unlike most human prescriptions. In other words, I'd have to examine your raccoon. This is important. You and your children may be in danger—"

"I'm sorry," she said before I could finish. "I do not want to bring him in. I know you'll take him away from us." And she hung up again.

Three days later came the final call, and now she sounded really frightened.

"Doctor Metz, please help me. My baby raccoon is having fits. I'm so frightened—he's been sleeping with my children."

By now my frustration with this lady had reached the boiling point. I said, "Listen carefully. For the sake of your children's lives, bring that raccoon down to my office now!" Within ten minutes, the pathetic little creature was in my hospital in a picnic basket. The woman stood in my reception room asking, "What are you going to do, Dr. Metz?"

Fortunately, her children were not there to hear my answer, which was, "I now have no choice. We must be sure this raccoon does not have rabies. That means we have to put the poor little one to sleep." What I didn't tell her was that if the raccoon tested positive for rabies, both she and her children would probably have to undergo the whole series of post exposure anti-rabies injections. Thankfully, this little raccoon did not have rabies. He did have canine distemper—quite common in urban and suburban raccoons. This is usually a fatal disease for raccoons and dogs, but it is not communicable to humans.

In each of the preceding three stories, I was asked for advice, I gave the best advice I could, and it was ignored, with real or potential harm as the result. This type of scenario is not unique to my practice. If almost any physician or veterinarian were asked, "What is the most vexing problem that must be dealt with in medical practice?" the most common answer would almost certainly be patient or client compliance.

For the most part, the people with whom I've had a doctor-client relationship during my years of practice have been honest and trustworthy, if not always agreeable. However, as I've already noted, there are times when an owner's perception of their own responsibility toward their pet differs greatly

Steven B. Metz, d.v.m.

from that of the veterinarian. Here is one of the most egregious examples of this conflict and the result of it.

On an early spring evening, before the existence of the regional emergency hospital, I took a call from a young lady who said she didn't have a regular veterinarian, but that her female cat had just been hit by a car and didn't seem to be able to use her hind legs. She also made sure to tell me that she had no way to pay for veterinary service. I asked if she had any family or friends who could help with the expenses. She said no, and seemed quite upset with me for asking about payment when her cat was injured.

At this point, then, I had to make a basic decision. Here was a person I had never seen before. She had no regular veterinarian who might have helped her based on his or her past relationship. My chances of being paid for the emergency service didn't seem good. Unlike human medicine, there is no law that requires me to see any patient. Financial difficulties can happen to any pet owner, but most people seem to accept the premise that one cannot walk into any place of business as a stranger and demand service without expecting to pay for it. Most pet owners at least try to make some sort of financial arrangements if an emergency occurs, but this young lady dismissed any suggestion I made, and did so with no apology.

Realizing that this emergency visit might end up being a total gift, I told the owner to bring her cat to my hospital. When she arrived (driving a late model automobile in good condition, I observed), I found out the following information: this cat had never been to a veterinarian, had never had any vaccinations, and was not spayed; she had just had a litter of four kittens (left at home); and the owner lived on a busy street in Burlington. The cat was kept on an open porch outside—she was rarely in the house, even with kittens.

"I don't like indoor litter boxes," the owner told me. "Besides, she wants to be outside. She likes to hunt."

I didn't ask her what she thought her cat was hunting on the streets of Burlington. Instead, I carefully examined the cat, noting that she was breathing easily, the color of her gums and tongue were pink, and her heart and lungs sounded quite normal. Her abdomen felt relaxed and was not painful. She could bear weight on her front legs, and could move, but could not support any weight on her back legs. She also had normal feeling in the back legs. There were a few minor scrapes on each back paw, but no other wounds or detectable injuries.

The most likely reason for this cat's inability to support on her back legs was a fractured pelvis. This diagnosis could only be confirmed by radiography.

Although obviously uncomfortable, neither this nor any other injury the kitty had sustained was immediately life threatening.

"Here is what I will do for you and your cat," I told the owner. "I will treat and bandage the wounds on her paws, and I'll give you some pain medication for her for the next few days. However, I will not x-ray her until you can help me with the cost of her treatment." This approach seemed quite reasonable to me. In fact I felt it was generous, considering the circumstance. But it did not satisfy this young lady.

"You're going to let my cat suffer with a broken pelvis on account of money? What kind of a veterinarian are you? You are supposed to love animals and take care of them. That's your job," she lectured me. I confess to becoming very angry when I heard that.

I said, "What about your job? This is your cat. You are responsible. You have no right to expect me to lend you money to take care of your obligations."

There was more of this heated exchange—none of which, of course, resulted in a better understanding. In the end, she left the hospital with her cat nestled on a soft absorbent blanket in a carrier, both of which I gave her, along with medication for pain and instructions to make sure she was eating, drinking, and eliminating normally. I reiterated that I would be happy to pursue further diagnostics and treatment the minute she could help with the cost. It was no surprise that she wasn't a bit curious to know the cost of the emergency care I had given, nor did she thank me in any way for coming in at night to take care of her cat. It was likewise no surprise that I never heard from her again.

In addition to this disheartening type of experience, there have been a few times when an owner has deliberately given me false information in hopes that I would find something to justify a more desirable outcome for a problem. Thus, Robert, a local breeder of golden retrievers, brought in a two-year-old male dog with the complaint that he wasn't moving well and seemed to fatigue very easily when retrieving. The physical examination all seemed normal, so I took a blood sample to check liver and kidney function, white and red blood cell counts, and also to make sure this dog did not have heartworm, since fatigue is perhaps the most common sign of that disease.

All the blood results were normal for the young dog, and to my surprise, Robert suggested taking films of the dog's hips and rear end. I was surprised because it was usually pretty difficult to persuade Robert to spend money on diagnostic tests. I readily agreed to doing the radiographs. After all, this dog could have hip dysplasia, an inherited malformation of the hip joints. When I

Steven B. Metz, d.v.m.

took and read the films, however, I got an unpleasant shock. This dog's rear was full of small birdshot! Someone had shot this dog and at close range to boot. No wonder he wasn't moving well! In fact, the real wonder was that he could run at all, considering the load of shot he was carrying.

As I thought more about the situation, something didn't quite add up. There were no skin wounds where the birdshot had penetrated, which suggested that the shooting had occurred at least a few weeks before the visit. Why had Robert not discovered that his dog had been shot when it first happened? I told Robert about the birdshot and showed him the films. He seemed surprised, but not outraged, as I would have expected any dog owner to be when he found out that his dog had been shot.

I dispensed anti-inflammatory pain medication, and the dog's gait gradually got better over the next few months. It wasn't until almost a year later, when I happened to meet Robert at a grocery store, that he told me the truth about the young dog with the birdshot in his rear end.

He, himself, had shot his own dog! He had read in some sporting magazine that if you were training a retriever to follow whistle or hand signals and the dog wasn't paying proper attention, the trainer should shoot the dog's rear. From then on, apparently, the dog would pay strict attention. Robert had known, then, what the problem was when he brought the dog in to see me, but he wanted to see just how badly he'd hurt his dog. Needless to say, I was so disgusted with Robert and his "training methods" that I had very little to do with him from that time on.

We have seen some examples in which there was no happy ending and the outcome was not favorable to the pet involved. Here is an episode where everything did turn out well, in spite of a bad start—an episode that, by the way, could have landed me in jail.

On a Labor Day holiday weekend, I happened to be at the hospital checking on a patient when the doorbell rang and in walked a middle-aged woman carrying an Old English sheepdog puppy. Tears were streaming down her face. My first thought was that the puppy had been hit by a car or suffered some other terrible accident. I rushed over and took the puppy from the woman's arms, and before she could even say anything, I quickly examined the puppy's gums, which were nice and pink, and I put a stethoscope on the pup's chest to listen to the heart and lungs, which sounded perfectly normal.

"No, no," said the woman, "That's not the problem. He's blind!"

I looked at the puppy's eyes, and it was obvious that this little doggie had juvenile cataracts involving the lenses of both eyes. Juvenile cataracts are an inherited condition that shows up at a young age and depending on the severity of the cataracts, can mean that the affected puppy will be completely or partially blind all its life.

I could understand why the woman was upset, but this was not exactly an emergency situation. Why, then, had she rushed into the hospital so frantically? I calmed her down as much as I was able, and this is the story she told me.

She had come to Burlington that morning from the Montreal, Quebec area because she had always wanted an Old English sheepdog, and she had seen an advertisement in a Montreal newspaper listing a litter of puppies for sale. She called the phone number listed in the ad and spoke with the "breeder" who said that he had one puppy left. He told the woman he had been saving this puppy because it was the pick of the litter, and he was considering keeping it and showing the puppy himself. All of that, of course, made her more anxious to have this puppy. Thus, she arranged to meet the "breeder" in the parking lot of a Burlington area supermarket. He couldn't invite her to his kennels, he said, because he was on his way out of town.

She met the man in the parking lot. She said he seemed quite disheveled and was in a hurry. He said he would mail her the registration papers along with his business card (he'd forgotten his business cards, he said). She liked the looks of the puppy, she did not bother to get any sort of health guarantee, and she paid this man $450 in U.S. cash. Fortunately, she insisted on a receipt, which he wrote out on a piece of scrap paper.

It may be easy for us, looking through the "retrospectoscope" to ask why the woman went along with this unsavory way of acquiring a puppy. If we put ourselves in her place, however, it becomes more understandable. She was not an experienced dog owner, she knew no one in the area, the man had built up the puppy over the phone, and then she actually held the puppy—which she had wanted for so long—all this was an undeniable combination of circumstances.

Unfortunately, this woman was dealing with the most infamous professional con man in the greater Burlington area. This man was well known by all the veterinarians and reputable dog breeders—we had attempted, time after time, to put this fellow out of business and to prosecute him for unscrupulous business practices. But he knew all the twists and loopholes in the law, and no one so far had been able to prove wrongdoing that would stand up in court.

I, myself, had had dealings with this man when I x-rayed the hip joints of one of his dogs, and he tried to get me to sign a certificate saying the films were

STEVEN B. METZ, D.V.M.

those of another dog. He also sold a puppy in my hospital parking lot, and when the purchaser insisted on a veterinary exam as part of the deal, he came into the examination room and nervously tried to tone down everything I noticed about this skinny little puppy he was selling—fleas, ear mites, and almost certainly, intestinal parasites. That was the last time I had anything to do with him until this Labor Day weekend.

I was outraged by the way this predator had used the Canadian woman's desire for a puppy of this breed to sell her a blind dog without telling her anything about the cataracts. Although it was a Sunday and a holiday, I picked up the phone and called my attorney, Peter Collins, the second person I met when I first came to Vermont in 1972. He had become a good friend as well as my attorney, and I felt the circumstances warranted drastic action. His wife said he was out on his sailboat, moored at the Lake Champlain Yacht Club not far from my office. I put the woman and her puppy in my car and drove out to the Yacht Club. From the shore, I could see Peter moving around on his boat, but even calling as loud as I could, I wasn't able to get his attention. There didn't seem to be anyone around who could give me a ride out to his boat, so in desperation, I jumped into a rowboat tied up at the dock—I had no idea whose boat it was—and rowed out to Peter's boat. He was surprised to see me.

"I didn't know you had a boat out here," he said.

"I don't. I just sort of borrowed this one for a minute. I have a legal emergency, Peter," I said.

"Uh oh," he said. "What did you do?" I quickly filled him in on the puppy scam.

"I know where this crook lives and I have his telephone numbers," I told Peter. "Will you come to my office with me to help me threaten him legally? Maybe we can get this lady's money back if we throw a good scare into him. Besides that, if the owner of this boat comes back and finds it missing, you'll have another job on your hands—defending me against charges of theft!"

At that, Peter jumped into his little outboard skiff, I got back in my borrowed rowboat, and we both went back to the Yacht Club. Fortunately, no one seemed to be concerned about a missing boat.

Our Canadian victim was waiting with her blind puppy, and I introduced her to Peter. I could see that, being a dog owner himself, he was entirely sympathetic to the idea of getting the con artist to return the money paid for this pup. We drove back to the hospital, and I got the man on the telephone. With Peter listening on another extension, I didn't mince any words.

"Listen carefully," I said. "I have the victim of your latest crooked dealings sitting right here in my office. I also have my attorney here listening to our conversation. You know very well that you sold her a blind puppy, one that you completely misrepresented as the pick of the litter. I don't like to threaten anyone, but I expect you to come down to my office immediately and return this woman's money. The arrangements you make concerning this poor puppy are between you and our Canadian visitor, but you will not charge her one cent for this dog if she wants to keep the pup. My attorney is not sitting here for his own amusement. I'm sure I don't have to say any more."

There was a moment of silence at the other end of the line, then the man said, "I had no idea the puppy was blind."

"I absolutely do not believe you. But that doesn't matter. You will return the money right now," I said. And that is exactly what happened. Peter typed up a letter releasing the puppy's owner (it turned out that she wanted to keep him) from any claims by this pseudo-breeder con artist. He came to the office, returned the money, signed the release, didn't even quibble about the puppy staying with the woman he'd cheated, and drove off. I never saw him again.

The blind puppy's new owner went back to Quebec, and later wrote me that with the help of a skillful trainer, she had trained the puppy to respond to whistle signals, and that on his own home territory, it was impossible to tell that he was blind.

As for Peter, he breathed a great sigh of relief that no violence had occurred (I had been very angry), and went back to the peace of his boat, hoping never again to suffer such an invasion of his privacy. We remain good friends to this day.

I sometimes marvel at my journey from being a boy who would have been frightened by even a fluffy, blind puppy on his walk to school to becoming a practicing veterinarian. Who would have imagined that between those early days and now I would have braved placing a needle in the tail of a tiger, looked an elephant in the eye, and set up a cot next to a client's sick Doberman to hold careful vigil. These many years have been spent helping people and their creature companions—be they domestic or exotic.

It has been an incredibly rich and fulfilling life. I owe my success, first and foremost, to my beloved grandfather who answered my preponderance of questions as a curious young boy, and to our family's boxer, Duke, who helped me overcome my crippling fear of animals. Thank you Grandpa Katzman, thank you Duke, and thank you to the many others who have been my faithful companions, my guides, and my teachers.

Epilogue

It would take a writer with far greater skills than I possess to sum up a career spanning almost forty-two years of companion and exotic animal veterinary practice. I have tried to include stories that represent some of the highlights. I could have included dozens more episodes in almost every chapter, each one unique in some way.

One morning a few years ago, I was preparing to go to the hospital for a full day of appointments when my eldest son Andrew, who was at the time a reporter for a New York newspaper, asked me, "Do you look forward to going to work every day?"

I answered him (as I have others who have asked me the same question), "Andrew, in all my years in this profession, I have never had a moment of regret. I have never been bored, and when I can help someone with a beloved pet in trouble, I feel the same thrill of accomplishment that I did at the very beginning."

Through my work I have been privileged to count as colleagues some of the most inspiring, dedicated people in my life. Many of these colleagues have become like family, sharing in the happy occasions as well as the sorrows of our lives. I can think of nothing more rewarding than to remain involved with my profession and my colleagues as long as I am physically and mentally able to do so. I can think of no life richer than mine has been, with family, friends, and colleagues, and the privilege of helping people realize the rewards that come with a life shared with the other creatures on our planet.

—*June 7, 2011, Cliff Island, Maine*

Acknowledgements

This book came to be written because frequently during my years of practice, my clients, my nurse/technicians, my friends, and even my colleagues, upon hearing the stories of some of my more unusual adventures, said to me, "You ought to write a book." As a result of these urgings, I began carrying a little pocket notebook with me during my appointment hours. I used it to jot down notations about cases and encounters that, perhaps, were not average, everyday companion animal experiences (if, indeed, there is such a thing).

First and foremost, I must thank my parents, my brother, my numerous aunts and uncles, and my beloved grandfather. Once they became resigned to the fact that I had no intention of becoming a "real doctor," they supported my efforts in every possible way, and they suffered along with me as I received rejection after rejection.

Much of my love for and appreciation of the natural world and its creatures came from a seventh grade science teacher, Miss Claudia Schmidt. Her ability to inspire the most unruly of students and to communicate the lure of the very discipline of the scientific method was a rare gift. More than sixty years later, I am left with gratitude for my good fortune in having shared part of my life with such a teacher.

My wife, Connie, has travelled with me from our mutual home in Springfield, Massachusetts to Alaska, to Canada, and back to New England on the quest to realize my dream of entering the veterinary profession. She lived through the same agonies of rejection and self doubt with me, and when the great day came for me to begin my professional education, she encouraged and supported me throughout the four years at Ontario Veterinary College, throughout my apprenticeship at the Warwick Animal Hospital, and took the gamble with me of giving up a secure position and starting a new practice in an area where neither of us had any friends or even acquaintances.

Our three children learned to cope with my irregular hours, and to accept my sleeping bag and x-ray table as a sick bed. All were supportive, if a little incredulous, about their veterinarian father actually writing a book.

I have devoted a chapter of this book to the remarkable professional education I received at the Ontario Veterinary College and the veterinary professors who "administered" it. I have tried to convey my respect and admiration for the patience and talent of these men and women, whose influence and inspiration persisted throughout my entire career.

I was fortunate beyond words that my first position as a graduate veterinarian resulted in the guidance of Drs. George Maurice and Jim Robbin at the Warwick Animal Hospital in Rhode Island, who showed me by personal example the heights of professional ethics and merit to which I aspired during my career. Their skill in teaching and their enthusiastic passion for their profession filled me from the first days of our association and is with me to this day.

Throughout my forty-one years of active veterinary practice, I was aided by many dedicated and talented veterinary nurse/technicians. This group of professionals has often been underappreciated by both veterinarians and pet owners. I believe I speak for most veterinarians when I say it would be extremely difficult to operate any type of veterinary practice without this well-educated, motivated element of the veterinary profession. I would particularly like to acknowledge and thank Linda Perrin and Alison Booth, my first two technicians—both of whom helped me begin practice, make many important, practice-shaping decisions, and faithfully helped me scrub the hospital floors every Sunday morning. The decision to retire from active practice was a difficult one for me; along with my family, I was supported by Shannon Wright, RVT—my last and most skilled technician. By challenging me to both teach and learn she made my final years in practice some of the most stimulating of my entire career. When the time came, she helped me leave active practice with relative grace.

I wrote most of this book while staying by the sea amongst the generous, welcoming residents of Cliff Island, Maine, who provided the peaceful environment that allowed me to write without being disturbed. I am especially grateful to Pam and Norman "Bub" Anderson and their son Eric, who unfailingly ministered to my passion for lobster and saw to my Maine education in general and Cliff Island protocols in particular. When the Andersons couldn't help, Billy O'Reilly and Joanne LaPomarda filled in with both lobsters and stories. Also, a fond thanks to Tom and Anne O'Reilly who welcomed me to Cliff Island one raw winter's evening with homemade chicken soup, and whose enthusiasm for life on the Island no matter the time of year or weather added to each of my stays. Perhaps the most patient of all Cliff Islanders is Chester Pettengill, owner and operator of the Island's taxi service. No matter what time of the day I arrived or departed, sometimes in rather uncomfortable weather, Chester faithfully and uncomplainingly helped transport my numerous bags and bundles to and from the ferry, which luggage ranged from live lobsters to dog food, along with the consumer of the dog food, my German shorthair, Bella.

Finally, to the staff of Wind Ridge Publishing, Inc., particularly to editors Emily Copeland and Lin Stone, for their extraordinary gentility and patience in helping me shape my words so as to allow me to communicate my thoughts and experiences clearly and rationally, I owe great thanks. Without their efforts, this book might never have become a reality.

The profession of veterinary medicine has often been glamorized to the point of distortion. Consequently, some people—especially those who love animals—are attracted to the profession only to be disillusioned after closer contact. Perhaps this book will take some of the mystery out of a career in veterinary medicine and be of use to students considering such a path.

CPSIA information can be obtained at www.ICGtesting.com
Printed in the USA
BVOW011643150712

295205BV00003B/2/P